"This book is a wonderful addition to the numerous volumes dealing with the work of Wilfred Bion. It offers a wide array of contributions and clinical illustrations written by an impressive international group of authors and will deepen the reader's understanding and breadth of Bion's writings. I highly recommend it to clinicians on all levels of training who are interested in the study of Bion's works and their application to psychoanalytic practice and theory."

Lawrence J. Brown, Ph.D, editor of *On Freud's Moses and Monotheism* (2023) and author of *Transformational Processes in Clinical Psychoanalysis* (2019)

"*The Bion Seminars at the A-Santamaría Association* is an enlightening and stimulating collection of chapters that delve deeply into the complexities of the human psyche as reflected in some of Wilfred Bion's most beautiful writings. Each chapter offers unique insights and perspectives that contribute to a comprehensive exploration of psychoanalytic theory and clinical practice. From the concept of the imaginary twin to negative capability and the concept of 'transformation,' this book navigates the intricacies of Bion's psychoanalysis with expertise and finesse. The contributors offer perspectives and intuitions that challenge conventional wisdom and expand our understanding of the human experience. Whether exploring Bion's issues about the limits of language or the meaning of frustration, these chapters invite readers on a journey that will leave them with a passionate picture of one of the most original and thought-provoking writers in the history of psychoanalysis. This book is a valuable resource for clinicians, researchers, and anyone in the field of humanities interested in what psychoanalysis can tell us about the essence of our humanity."

Giuseppe Civitarese, author of *Psychoanalytic Field Theory: A Contemporary Introduction* (2022)

The Bion Seminars at the A-Santamaría Association

The Bion Seminars at the A-Santamaria Association offers readers insightful analyses and commentaries on Bion's key papers and books, as well as providing a unique set of discussions and explorations of many of Bion's central concepts and foundational texts.

This diverse collection of essays brings together contributions from internationally renowned Bionian scholars and analysts, including Annie Reiner, Nicola Abel-Hirsch, Antònia Grimalt, Avner Bergstein, Afsaneh Kiany Alisobhani, João Carlos Braga, Tom Helscher, Tim Smith and Peter Goldberg. Readers will encounter expansions and extensions of contemporary and timeless themes and discover the originality with which psychoanalysts from different geographical regions take ownership of the ideas discussed. Chapters cover the early and late work of Bion, spanning topics such as arrogance, the theory of thinking, memory and desire, and the clinical importance of frustration. The authors reveal to us the elements of continuity and discontinuity in Bion's work, sharing open conjectures to allow new developments to evolve.

This volume is essential reading for practicing psychoanalysts, analysts-in-training, analytic psychotherapists, and anyone interested in exploring Bion's work.

Howard B. Levine is a member of APSA, PINE, the Contemporary Freudian Society and Pulsion; he is on the faculty of NYU Post-Doc's Contemporary Freudian Track, on the editorial boards of the *International Journal of Psychoanalysis* and *Psychoanalytic Inquiry*, editor-in-chief of the Routledge Wilfred Bion Studies Book Series and in private practice in Brookline, Massachusetts, USA.

Jani Santamaría Linares is a member of APSA, APM, FEPAL, IPA and the International Advisory Committee of the Routledge Bion Studies Book Series, director of A-Santamaría Psychoanalysis Mexico A.C., a training and supervising analyst for children and adolescents, a member of the International Committee of Spanish Language Psychoanalysts and in private practice in Mexico City.

The Routledge Wilfred R. Bion Studies Book Series
Series Editor
Howard B. Levine, MD

The contributions of Wilfred Bion are among the most cited in the analytic literature. Their appeal lies not only in their content and explanatory value, but in their generative potential. Although Bion's training and many of his clinical instincts were deeply rooted in the classical tradition of Melanie Klein, his ideas have a potentially universal appeal. Rather than emphasizing a particular psychic content (e.g., Oedipal conflicts in need of resolution; splits that needed to be healed; preconceived transferences that must be allowed to form and flourish, etc.), he tried to help open and prepare the mind of the analyst (without memory, desire or theoretical preconception) for the encounter with the patient.

Bion's formulations of group mentality and the psychotic and non-psychotic portions of the mind, his theory of thinking and emphasis on facing and articulating the truth of one's existence so that one might truly learn first hand from one's own experience, his description of psychic development (alpha function and container/contained) and his exploration of O are "non-denominational" concepts that defy relegation to a particular school or orientation of psychoanalysis. Consequently, his ideas have taken root in many places.... and those ideas continue to inform many different branches of psychoanalytic inquiry and interest.[1]

It is with this heritage and its promise for the future developments of psychoanalysis in mind that we present *The Routledge Wilfred Bion Studies Book Series*. This series gathers together under newly emerging and continually evolving contributions to psychoanalytic thinking that rest upon Bion's foundational texts and explore and extend the implications of his thought. For a full list of titles in the series, please visit the Routledge website at: https://www.routledge.com/The-Routledge-Wilfred-Bion-Studies-Book-Series/book-series/RWBSBS

Howard B. Levine, MD
Series Editor

1   Levine, H.B. and Civitarese, G. (2016). Editors' Preface, *The W.R. Bion Tradition*, Levine and Civitarese, eds., London: Karnac 2016, p. xxi.

The Bion Seminars at the A-Santamaría Association

Clinical and Theoretical Explorations

Edited by
Howard B. Levine and Jani Santamaría
Linares

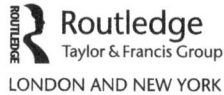

Routledge
Taylor & Francis Group

LONDON AND NEW YORK

Designed cover image: © Claude Monet, Poppy Field at Giverny

First published 2025
by Routledge
4 Park Square, Milton Park, Abingdon, Oxon OX14 4RN

and by Routledge
605 Third Avenue, New York, NY 10158

Routledge is an imprint of the Taylor & Francis Group, an informa business

British Library Cataloguing-in-Publication Data
A catalogue record for this book is available from the British Library

ISBN: 978-1-032-66121-6 (hbk)
ISBN: 978-1-032-64164-5 (pbk)
ISBN: 978-1-032-66123-0 (ebk)

DOI: 10.4324/9781032661230

Typeset in Times New Roman
by Taylor & Francis Books

With all my love, I dedicate this book to my son José Luis for his patience and for being a life miracle that inspires me to be more than I can be.

Jani Santamaría Linares

Contents

Contributors

Nicola Abel-Hirsch is a training and supervising analyst of the British Psycho-analytical Society. She has given theoretical and clinical papers on Bion in the UK, Taiwan (annually, 2005–2012), the USA, and Europe. She is the editor of Hanna Segal's last book, *Yesterday, Today and Tomorrow* (2007), and the author of *Bion 365 Quotes* (2019) and *Bion: An Introduction (2023)*. She leads an ongoing series of seminars on Bion's thought and work under the auspices of Understanding Primitive Mental States, New York City.

Afsaneh Kiany Alisobhani is a training and supervising psychoanalyst at the Newport Psychoanalytic Institute (NPI) and a member of the faculty at the New Center for Psychoanalysis in Los Angeles (NCP). She is an associate clinical professor at the Department of Psychiatry and Human Behavior, School of Medicine, University of California. She was the co-chair of the International Bion Conference in Los Angeles in 2014 and the co-editor of *Exploration in Bion's 'O': Everything We Know Nothing About*, published by Routledge in 2020.

Avner Bergstein is a training and supervising analyst and faculty member of the Israel Psychoanalytic Society. He works in private practice with adults, adolescents, and children and has worked for several years at a kindergarten for children with autism. He has authored numerous papers elaborating on the clinical implications of the writings of Bion and Meltzer and is the author of the book *Bion and Meltzer's Expeditions into Unmapped Mental Life: Beyond the Spectrum in Psychoanalysis* (Routledge, 2018). He is a visiting lecturer at several psychoanalytic institutes and conducts reading seminars focusing on the writings of W.R. Bion. In 2021, he received the IPA's Elizabeth Young-Bruehl Prejudice Award.

João Carlos Braga is a graduate in medicine from the Federal University of Paraná, Brazil (1966) and was a fellow at Baylor University, Department of Psychiatry, Houston, Texas (1967). He is currently a member of the faculty and a training and supervising analyst at the Brazilian

Psychoanalytic Society of São Paulo and the Curitiba Psychoanalytic Society. He has published approximately 30 psychoanalytical papers and book chapters in various books and in national and international journals.

Peter Goldberg is a personal and supervising analyst at the Psychoanalytic Institute of Northern California (PINC), chair of faculty at the San Francisco Center for Psychoanalysis, on the faculty of the Wright Institute in Berkeley, and is co-author of *Here I Am Alive: The Spirit of Music in Psychoanalysis* (Columbia University Press, 2023).

Antònia Grimalt is a training and supervising analyst of the Spanish Society (SEP-IPA) and of FEAP, a former chair of the Forum for Child Psychoanalysis (FEP), a child and adolescent training analyst of EPI (the former Hans Groen Prakken Institute), a teacher of Klein and Bion in two university master's degree programs, and the director of many seminars about Klein and Bion at the SEP Institute, including one about *A Memoir of the Future*. As a member of the Ed. Monografies de Psicoanàlisi i Psicoteràpia, she has been translating books about Bion into Catalan, is editor of the complete works of Pere Folch, editor of the very first Catalan translation of *Bion in Los Angeles*, the Spanish edition of Matte Blanco's *Thinking, Feeling and Being*, and editor of the Catalan edition of Ricardo Lombardi's *Formless Infinity*. She was also chair of the 2020 International Bion Conference: Intuition held in Barcelona.

Thomas Helscher is a training and supervising analyst at LAISPS and on the faculty at LAISPS and WILA. He has written and presented on transgenerational transmission of trauma, on moral injury as an alternative to PTSD, and on the frame in psychoanalysis. He is in private practice in Los Angeles, CA.

Howard B. Levine is a member of APSA, PINE, the Contemporary Freudian Society and Pulsion, on the faculty of NYU Post-Doc's Contemporary Freudian Track, on the editorial board of the *International Journal of Psychoanalysis* and *Psychoanalytic Inquiry*, editor-in-chief of the Routledge Wilfred Bion Studies book series, and in private practice in Brookline, Massachusetts. He is the author of *Transformations de l'Irreprésentable* (Ithaque, 2019) and *Affect, Representation and Language: Between the Silence and the Cry* (Routledge, 2022) and editor of *The Post-Bionian Field Theory of Antonino Ferro* (Routledge, 2022), *The Freudian Matrix of Andre Green. Towards a Psychoanalysis for the 21st Century* by André Green (Routledge/IPA, 2023), and André Green's *On The Destruction and Death Drives* (Phoenix/Karnac, 2023). His co-edited books include *Unrepresented States and the Construction of Meaning* (Karnac, 2013), *On Freud's Screen Memories* (Karnac, 2014), *The Wilfred Bion Tradition* (Karnac, 2016), *Bion in Brazil* (Karnac, 2017), *The Clinical Thinking of W.R. Bion in Brazil* (Routledge, 2024),

André Green Revisited: Representation and the Work of the Negative (Karnac, 2018), *Covidian Life* (2021, Phoenix), *Psychoanalysis of the Psychoanalytic Frame Revisited: A New Look at Bleger's Classical Work* (Routledge/IPA, 2022), *On the Destruction and Death Drives by André Green* (Phoenix, 2023), and *Autistic Phenomena and Unrepresented States: Explorations in the Emergence of Self* (Phoenix, 2023).

Annie Reiner is a senior faculty member and training analyst at the Psychoanalytic Center of California (PCC) in Los Angeles. Her work was greatly influenced by Wilfred Bion, with whom she studied in the 1970s. She lectures around the world, is published in numerous journals and anthologies, and is the author of four psychoanalytic books, including *The Quest for Conscience & The Birth of the Mind* (Karnac, 2009), *Bion and Being: Passion and the Creative Mind* (Karnac, 2012), *Of Things Invisible to Mortal Sight: Celebrating the Work of James S. Grotstein* (Karnac, 2017), and, most recently, *W.R. Bion's Theories of Mind: A Contemporary Introduction* (Routledge, 2022). She is also a poet, painter, and singer and, in addition to her psychoanalytic writings, she is the author of a book of short stories, four books of poems, and six children's books, which she also illustrated. She supervises and maintains a psychoanalytic practice in Beverly Hills, California.

Jani Santamaría Linares is a training analyst and supervisor of children, adolescents and adults of the Mexican Psychoanalytic Association (APM), director of the A. Santamaría Psychoanalysis Mexico A.C. Educational Association, and on the International Advisory Committee of the Routledge W.R. Bion Studies book series. She is a former Latin-American board member of the International Psychoanalytic Association (IPA) (2019–2021/ 2021–2023). She is a member of the American Psychoanalytic Association (APsA) and was chair of the International Bion Conference Mexico City, 2022, chair of the Latin-American Winnicott Congress, Mexico City, 2017, and former director of community and culture for FEPAL (2016–2018). She is a member of the International Committee of Spanish Language Psychoanalysts. She is co-author of *Autistic Phenomena and Unrepresented States: Explorations in the Emergence of Self* (Phoenix Publishing House, 2023), editor of *Bion, Dreamwork and the Oneiric Dimensions of the Mind* (Routledge, 2024, forthcoming), editor of 'Jugando con el Pensamiento de Winnicott en America Latina' (Ediciones Biebel, 2023), and editor of 'Virtualidad, Duelos y Migraciones en el Covid 19. Perspectivas Psicoanalíticas' (Ediciones Biebel, 2023). She has authored many national and international articles, book chapters, and reviews and has a private practice of child and adult psychoanalysis in Mexico City.

Tim Smith is a child and adolescent psychotherapist and member of the Association of Child and Adolescent Psychotherapists in the UK. He works for the National Health Service and is in private practice in East London.

Introduction

Jani Santamaría Linares

In July 1997, Parthenope Bion organized the first International Bion Conference in Torino, Italy, to celebrate the centennial of her father's birth (September 8, 1997). This experience started a tradition that turned into a forum to keep Bion's ideas alive and to build on and continue to elaborate his thoughts. It was in the spirit of this tradition that A-Santamaría Psychoanalysis Mexico A.C., a non-profit, independent psychoanalytic educational association, began organizing the first Mexican International Bion Conference, which was to be held in 2022. The initial plan of inviting outstanding scholars to offer a series of seminars that engaged with the full range of Bion's writings was interrupted by the presence of an uncomfortable and unexpected guest that impeded the continuity of this project. Just at the beginning of the seminar proposal, the COVID-19 pandemic struck. From the beginning, the coronavirus announced its invisible omnipresence and noisiness by inhabiting every particle of the universe. We were invaded intrusively by a deadly, volatile virus that had no nationality, no color, no taste, did not respect social class or protect human nature, knew no borders or containment walls, and passed over ethnicities, religions, and political systems, and, despite being the work of nature, not even God himself could stop it.

In Bion's *War Memoirs* (1997), it is to the fatal and bloody battle of Amiens, on August 8, 1918, that Bion most often refers, and he continued to return to it in his thoughts for the rest of his life (Abel-Hirsch 2023, p. 5). The tank he had been in was blown up by the enemy. He grabbed the belt of Sweeting, his runner, and pulled them both into a shell hole. Then, he realized that Sweeting was horribly wounded in the chest. The dramatic scene in which the dying Sweeting desperately asks Bion to please get in touch with his mother came to my mind as a paradigm of the deep need that every human being has for a containment function and another mind to help face the agonies of mortality and human existence. As Sweeting lay dying, Bion lay on the frozen ground and fantasized being held in his mother's arms (Bion 1997).

This heartbreaking scene also exemplifies what Bion meant by "thinking under fire". The same expression is also helpful to describe the experience of COVID-19, in which we were forced to 'think under COVID-19' in our 'trenches' (isolation), while the virus was raging around us. At this point, it is

DOI: 10.4324/9781032661230-1

unnecessary to describe once again the complicated and painful moments we have gone through. There is nothing more accurate than Bion's phrase to illustrate what most of us lived during those years: "Well, here we are … But where is here?" (Bion 1980, p. 9).

The need to contain this pandemic experience ignited the Diogenes lantern in our work as thinkers about mental states. During this humanitarian catastrophe, I asked myself how to transform the violence and helplessness of the moment into emotional growth and, at the same time, how to build a scientific bridge to keep the torch of the International Bion Conference Mexico 2022 alive. As an answer to the turbulence, and following Winnicott's idea that creativity means celebrating the fact of being alive, the Bion seminars moved to an online modality. The objective, which is now reflected in this book, was to approach Bion's work through the thoughts of a group of outstanding and distinguished international contributors from different geographical regions.

The originality of Bion's writings on the workings of the mind and its functions has opened up an enormous variety of avenues for exploration. His thinking is so rich, articulate, and complex that any attempt to clarify and develop it would be helpful. Therefore, discussions of his papers focusing on the clinical and theoretical implications of a particular approach to his thought and its possible developments would be even more relevant. This book of Bion seminars reflects deeply committed, solid contributions that center on understanding the essence of Bion's work.

As Grotstein wrote, Bion's ideas are highly unique and are presented by him with such density at times that it is often difficult to capture his meaning. "His published works remind me of solving a picture puzzle but one puzzle in which the configurations change as one is trying to find the right piece" (2007, p, 9). In that spirit, we invite you to read this book in the light of the concept of *caesura*. The chapters, as caesuras, can be read as gates where it is possible to be in contact with many branches of his thought and through which one can make contact with a language of achievement that can penetrate multiple chapters in an enlarging and evolving spiral of ideas. In this introduction, I will limit myself to briefly pointing out some glimpses of thought to stimulate curiosity and sustain the mystery of the content of each chapter.

Early Bion

The book begins with Tim Smith's paper, "Reading the Child and Adolescent Bion". This chapter describes the child and adolescent states of mind pertaining to adolescence and sexuality recalled by the eighty-year-old Bion in his autobiography *The Long Weekend 1897–1919: Part of a Life* (1982).

Bion's autobiographical narratives, *A Memoir of the Future* (1977a, 1979) and *The Long Week-End* (1982), together with the sequel, *All My Sins Remembered* (1985), are the key to his self-analysis. "Bion makes clear that the 'war' itself is simply the continuation of a pre-existing state of affairs, *ad absurdum*: 'schoolboys of all ages playing soldiers, rehearsing for the real thing, but never learning that war and yet more terrible war is normal, not an aberrant disaster'" (Harris Williams 2010). Many authors, such as Abel-Hirsch (2023), Bleandonu (1993) and Grotstein (2007), among others, have written about Bion's biography. Lawrence Brown (2012), for instance, wrote that Bion went through a personal process of thinking about his own traumatic experiences while, at the same time, formulating his concepts of alpha function and container–contained.

In a clear and concise way, Smith pays attention to the following points: the development of maturation and masculinity in young boys as seen from a psychoanalytic perspective; the forced separation of young British boys from their parents in the Edwardian era and the destructive impact this had on Bion's developing masculine identity; and the process of trauma on the lives of young men prior to World War I, especially in Britain. Smith (2021), who has been interested in the varied states of mind that Bion recalled in his autobiography about his childhood, adolescence, and young adulthood, argues that *The Long Weekend* is a seminal psychoanalytic autobiography and therefore a reliable source which takes the reader on a journey towards witnessing intimate truths.

Smith also describes a process of his own personal *reverie* that helped release further layers of meaning of Bion's descriptions of his child and adolescent states. He keenly explores how early traumatic experiences helped shape Bion's attitudes and approach to effective clinical work and how Bion's personal qualities of courage, his capacity to observe, and his interest in truth helped to counterbalance the destructiveness that had led him to reject close personal relationships. While *The Long Weekend* may prove difficult and demanding reading for some, Smith reminds us that, forty years after its original publication, it still has much to say about the nature of adolescent states of mind.

Bion's ideas, which could not have existed without Klein or Freud, brought a new paradigm to psychoanalysis beyond the scope of those earlier writers. In *Second Thoughts* (1967b), he brought together eight papers that represented an ongoing chronicle of his psychoanalytic work with psychotic patients and enriched our understanding of the communication process between the mind of the patient and analyst. In Chapters 2–4, the authors review articles produced in the 1950s – Bion's so-called early period – as they seek to follow the development of Bion's clinical thought and explore the foundations of his expansion of our understanding of the psychic apparatus proposed by Freud and implied by Klein's concept of projective identification.

In Chapter 2, Peter Goldberg explores Bion's paper "On Arrogance" (1958) and testifies to Bion's originality and clinical acumen. Goldberg points out that this paper manages to incite in the reader the intense curiosity that the paper warns us of and reminds us of the dilemma posed by the destructive potential inherent in the analytic pursuit of knowledge and truth at all costs.

Goldberg also explores several of Bion's highly original ideas: the identification of an underlying psychotic structure in otherwise apparently neurotic
patients, describing what might be called a post-catastrophic personality; the
way the analyst's curiosity and search for knowledge and understanding can
recapitulate the patient's experience of being disastrously impinged upon and
misunderstood; how the analyst, in his or her potentially arrogant search for
knowledge, can become the incarnation of an "obstructive object" that
cannot absorb or receive the patient's distress but, instead, exacerbates this
distress; and the implications of this for analytic practice – how we must
recognize the potential for destructive curiosity in our clinical approach and
must reposition ourselves to be receptive to the patient's 'primitive' modes of
communication, while avoiding arrogantly imposing our own way of knowing
and communicating upon the patient.

The paper ends with the recommendation that, in reading this article, the
best we can hope for is that our pride in ourselves and our work does not
curdle into arrogance, as Bion suggests it can, and that we try to remain
humble and willing to identify with the patient's suffering, legitimizing self-
respect, which also entails respect for others.

Second Thoughts (Bion 1967b) brought new ideas to the understanding of
psychosis but also, more importantly, laid the foundations for Bion's theory of
thinking. After Klein's death in 1960, Bion then set out his distillation of
what he had learned from both Klein and Freud, laying the groundwork for
his epistemological project. In "The Theory of Thinking" paper, as well as his
monograph *Learning from Experience* (1962a, 1962b), Bion tried to explicate
how the minds operates. He developed a highly creative theory of the mind
centered on the idea that the development of thoughts requires an apparatus
to cope with them. An expansion of these ideas is presented in Chapter 3, in
Tom Helscher's paper, "A Theory of Thinking".

Helscher begins this chapter by contextualizing "A Theory of Thinking",
saying that the paper constitutes perhaps Bion's most widely cited work, and
yet, like all of his writing, the deceptive simplicity of its premise belies the
complex depths it contains and the strange and surprising movement of its
line of argument.

He reminds us that this paper, one of the ten most cited psychoanalytic
papers on PEP, is deeply saturated with readings, interpretations, and layers
of meaning and is itself almost an institution or museum piece in the psychoanalytic literature. He therefore invites us to reread this paper without
memory, desire or understanding, so that we can experience it with new eyes.

According to Bion, the infant is born with a set of templates, called preconceptions, that are in search of 'realizations' through actual experience.
'Thought', which Bion differentiates from, and says precedes, 'thinking', is the
product of the mating of a preconception with a frustration. For Bion,
thoughts are the non-sensuous manifestation of the experience of frustration
that somehow emerges from the sensuous experience of pain, if we can bear

it. What makes thinking possible is the experience of the infant with another, an experience ('realization') of two-ness that opens the way to 'modification' of frustration rather than its denial. So, at the heart of this process of the development of thinking is a person's relation to the experience of frustration.

Helscher suggests that it is the ability of the infant or the immature aspects of the personality to experience two-ness characteristic of projective identification that allows for "the development of conceptions" in the absence of satisfying experience. This experience provides the satisfaction of mental or emotional containment that is analogous to the bodily satisfaction of digesting real milk. This distinction is critical, because, for Helscher, Bion is suggesting that the non-sensuous 'satisfaction' of mental containment is in some ways analogous or equivalent to the physiological satisfaction of a good feed, but in a different register. That is, it is the emotional containment (C–c) and not the experience of physiological satisfaction that lies at the origins of thinking.

By eschewing clinical examples in his essay, Bion forces us to experience some degree of frustration in our reading and thinking through process, thereby inviting us to generate our own penumbra of associations to his discourse from our clinical experience.

Helscher gives Bion's paper new life, expands upon it, and innovatively integrates it with much of Bion's other work. The results are exciting. He expertly balances profound and extensive scholarship with sound reasoning and with a reader-friendly style. In my opinion, this is one of the finest and most useful explanations of a paper that represents a major turning point in Bion's psychoanalytic episteme.

Interspersed in his writings on psychosis between 1954 and 1959, Bion returned to Freud's earlier formulations on the nature of psychosis, before eventually centering his efforts on the implications of Freud's "Two Principles" paper. In the latter, Freud believed that contact with reality can, for some people under some conditions, be so unbearably painful that the contact itself must be broken off. However, working with a conceptual structure anchored in repression and related defense mechanisms, Freud was not able to fully describe the annihilation of reality that characterizes psychotic experience. This is where Bion took Freud more than a step forward. He argued that dread and hatred of reality lead not only to attacks on the external world and the objects contained within it, but also to attacks on our capacity to experience reality at all.

Chapter 4, Afsaneh Kiany Alisobhani's paper, "Differentiation of the Psychotic from the Non-Psychotic Personality: A Link between Early and Late Bion", is an incredibly rich and generous contribution.

For Alisobhani, Bion, a Freudian at heart, wove together the "Formulations Regarding the Two Principles in Mental Functioning" and Melanie Klein's 1946 paper "Notes on Some Schizoid Mechanisms" into a creative model for understanding and working with psychosis.

The role of the drives, the preponderance of destructive impulses, the hatred of both internal and external reality, and the use of minute splitting and expulsion of the fragments of the apparatus of awareness of reality are explored in greater detail. Alisobhani also underscores Bion's methodology for observation and differentiated clinical management in contact with psychotic configurations. Bion's acute insight into psychotic states of mind has paved the way for developments that are far from exhausted.

Even though each paper in the collection published in *Second Thoughts* contains original ideas, all share common ideas that continue to be developed. Alisobhani (Chapter 4), for instance, suggests that Bion went on to develop the model of the container–contained from the relationship between the psychotic and the non-psychotic part of the mind. Furthermore, she affirms that the seeds of concepts such as the contact barrier, caesura, and K, L, and H links that he cultivated and developed in his later work were planted in this paper. She finishes her paper with the conviction that Bion's paper (1958) offers a profound insight into the complexities of the mind which he takes the next few decades to develop.

Perhaps Bion's best-known works are his four books from the 1960s: *Learning from Experience* (1962b), *Elements of Psychoanalysis* (1963), *Transformations* (1965), and *Attention and Interpretation* (1970). In his exploration of "thinking emotional experiences", Bion had developed a theory of thinking including concepts such as the contact barrier, alpha function, L, H, and K links, C–c, and PS-D, among others. For me, these concepts and the work of this period represent a critical bridge between Bion's conception of the way the mind works and the experiential level of the emotional psychoanalytic process.

At the core of *Learning from Experience* (1962a) is Bion's thinking about what he called "alpha function". Bion postulated that alpha function was the function in charge of transforming the baby's raw sensory primitive experience (the beta elements) into dreams and oneiric thoughts.

If beta elements – raw or fragmented experiences yet to be processed – are not contained by a person, they have to be evacuated. Once formed, alpha elements come to create the contact barrier that separates consciousness from the unconscious and are assembled, by "the apparatus for dreaming dreams" and "the apparatus for thinking thoughts", into the narrative bits that make up the chains of thoughts, conscious and unconscious. Alpha elements are necessary for emotional development regarding links (L, H, K) and determine the permeability of binocular vision and perspective reversal. As Helscher mentions in Chapter 3, the concepts of alpha function and maternal *reverie* are explored in "A Theory of Thinking".

Bion stressed the importance of the linking function between minds as the basis for psychic development and considered that an emotional experience cannot be conceived of in isolation from a relationship. In this realm, *reverie*, a state of mind, is defined as a factor of the mother's alpha function (Bion

1962a, p. 36). Bion's identification of *reverie* as a psychoanalytic concept has drawn attention to a dimension of the analyst's experience with tremendous potential to enrich our interpretive understanding.

While the groundwork for Bion's best known concept, container–contained, is laid in "On Arrogance" (1958), Goldberg insists that it is in *Attention and Interpretation* that Bion discusses the concept in more detail. This concept of container–contained lies at the heart of human development. The process of transformation is accomplished through alpha function, a capacity which has its roots in the early mother–infant relationship and by which mother gives meaning to the baby's purely emotional experiences. According to this formulation, the mother is receptive to the infant's projections of unmentalized beta elements and transforms these into alpha elements through her capacity for *reverie*. In this process, a state of fertile and emotionally growth-promoting relationship is produced.

Readings of early Bion and late Bion are experiences that stand in dialectical tension with one another. The two reflect different "vertices" (Bion 1970, p. 93) from which to view the analytic experience. They give stereoscopic depth to one another as opposed to simply succeeding or conversing with one another. Thus, readers of Chapters 1–4 will have access to Bion's contributions from his "early period" and should be prepared for the following chapters, which correspond to the 'late Bion'. The most polarizing of his ideas in this later period is the concept of O, which Bion considered to be the essential psychoanalytic perspective for doing clinical work.

Late Bion

"The Limitations of Language in the Psychic Realm" (Chapter 5), written by Annie Reiner, examines the role of language in the analytic situation and the challenges and opportunities of our having to resort to using language as a core medium of connection in our relationship with patients.

Bion discovered that, when we are confronted with the challenge of trying to fully convey or describe something about human life and emotional experience, we find ourselves up against the very limitations of language. In his commentary, Bion (1967a) laments his inability to truthfully convey the totality of his emotional experience in words. He is aware that the only description he can give is in terms appropriate to sensuous experience, although the experience also reflected psychic reality that is not representable by the words derived from sensuous reality.

Grounded in decades of clinical work, Reiner, who was a student of Bion's in the 1970s, echoes Bion's position and agrees that 'the facts' of psychoanalysis are invisible and immaterial facts that have no physical attributes. They cannot be seen, heard, touched, smelled, or tasted with the tongue. Discussions about language figure prominently in Bion's later ideas about metaphysical realities of the mind, about which he concluded that a new science of the mind was necessary. His proposal about O was his attempt to do so, but this would require of the analyst a peculiar state of mind. Bion's conception of the analytic state of mind (*reverie*) is one in which the analyst makes him- or herself as open as possible to experiencing what is true and attempts to find words to convey something of that truth to the patient.

Reiner succeeds in providing us with convincing clinical examples (Stella and Rache) of how to put these fine conceptual instruments to work creatively. In this regard, she demonstrates that the language of psychoanalysis is born of the moment in our relationship to each particular patient on each particular day. In this context, Reiner considers the concept of 'selected fact' as one of Bion's (1962a) most important and innovative clinical ideas, which she discusses in a masterly way, tracing the origins of O from its very beginnings in Bion's work on the selected fact and suggesting that hearing the selected fact depends upon the capacity for apprehending the intuitive waking dream state of the unknowable O.

In Chapter 6, "The Clinical Importance of Frustration", Nicola Abel-Hirsch introduces her understanding of Bion's 1962 choice to place the experience of frustration in mental life and in the psychoanalytical encounter at the heart of his model. Her clinical examples consider that both the patient and the analyst, including Bion himself, may be avoiding frustration.

She reminds us that, in "A Theory of Thinking" (1962a), Bion forces us to think about the relationship between the stimulus for thinking what he calls 'thoughts', and the pressure on the mind that thoughts create. The result is a continuum of possible responses, from evasion in the form of projection to tolerance in the form of modification of painful frustrations. Bion was particularly interested in the patient's attitude towards reality and the distinction between reality and measures taken to evade and modify it. Thus, Bion examined the vicissitudes of frustration tolerance as a central precondition for psychic development and the capacity for thought.

Abel-Hirsch also suggests that Bion had a 'military' response to frustration in which he attempts to unite with the people he is frustrated with against a common enemy. Examples are given from World War I, in which he mobilizes a group of men who were refusing to parade (the shared enemy is the 'Bosche'), and from World War II, where he joins together with the 'undisciplined' men in Northfield Military Hospital to fight against the shared enemy of 'neurosis'. Abel-Hirsch suggests that his writing about frustration is an attempt to induce his 'undisciplined' fellow analysts to join with him against the enemy of "memory and desire".

Last, but not least, in a moving vignette, Abel-Hirsch shows us again her theoretical creativity and clinical talent and her capacity to dialogue even with the most severe patients in a deeply human and inspired visionary way. Her clinical examples not only reflect her professional qualities and vast theoretical knowledge but also her skill in getting into a profound emotional contact with patients. They illustrate Bion's belief, begun some years before

("On Arrogance", 1958) in "intuition" as the required alternative to sense perception, a view that he later formulated in his own enigmatic, systematized way in *Attention and Interpretation*, published in 1970. In this book, he develops the theme of transformations in O further than he did in *Transformations* and he describes a different kind of psychoanalysis that requires a different frame of mind of the analyst than working with K.

In the next chapter, Chapter 7, Howard Levine conducts us through the masterpiece book, *Attention and Interpretation* (1970), noting that, in it, Bion contrasts the difference between two kinds of patients or states of mind: those who can, and those who cannot, stand to remain in contact with an anxiety-producing or frustrating reality long enough to tolerate and think about what, if anything, can be done about it, rather than reacting by trying to evade, deny, or distort the perception of the source of their frustration or displeasure. In so doing, Bion is amplifying and exploring Freud's (1911) "Two Principles of Mental Functioning" from a clinical vertex that investigates the vicissitudes of frustration tolerance. This inevitably leads to questions and considerations of existential experience, psychic representation, and the epistemological status of language, thought, and experience – that is, knowing (K) and being (O).

Levine goes on to discuss Bion's movement to a position of uncertainty, O, from the logical positivism and certainty of some contemporary Freudian and Kleinian thinking that was ultimately based on the drives as first cause. Levine's paper reflects an incredible capacity to widen his exploration of this book by linking Bion and Freud and tracing Bion's conceptual evolution in his lesser-known dialogue with the work of Freud. In so doing, he captures Bion's thinking at a unique moment of time in his theoretical and personal development and gives the reader an original glimpse into Bion's book.

In Chapter 8, "Memory and Desire", Antònia Grimalt introduces the reader to one of the main theoretical and technical features of contemporary psychoanalysis. Decades ago, Bion's presentation, and later the publication of this paper, caused quite a storm (Abel-Hirsch 2023, p. 81). Grimalt illustrates essential aspects of Bion's later thinking and clarifies one of Bion's most clinically relevant ideas: the value of suspending elements of our memory and desire to allow openness to the ineffable. She begins her chapter with a reference to T.S. Eliot's verse, which expresses how preexisting knowledge, especially knowledge based on preconceptions and repeated expectations, tends to falsify direct perception and observation and distort hope and love. Grimalt then explores the complex development of Freud's classic technical recommendation – free-floating attention. Bion starts from the consideration of two kinds of memory, accumulative and evocative or oneiric, and discusses the theoretical pillars that are the foundations of a discipline focused on the centrality of the emotional experience in the analytic link.

As Reiner pointed out previously, Bion (1970) also links O to the capacity to suspend memory, desire, and understanding, as "preparatory to a state of mind in which O can evolve" (p. 33). This difficult mental discipline helps the analyst to "become infinite" (Bion 1970, p. 46), allowing the analyst to come into contact with the essential experience of the session.

Chapter 9 is "Caesura: A Close Reading Seminar of Bion's Text", in which Avner Bergstein leads readers through the most significant vertices of Bion's caesura paper (1977b). He leans upon Freud's statement that "There is much more continuity between intra-uterine life and earliest infancy than the impressive caesura of the act of birth allows us to believe". Bion drew a totally new way of thinking from this passage as he made caesura a pivotal concept in his theories. What Bergstein aims at in his reading is underlining the different ways in which we can read this paper, and he proposes the caesura of birth as a metaphor for all that is concealed from us.

Bion's brave and daring notion of "caesura" suggests a link between mature emotions and thinking and intra-uterine life and serves as a model for bridging seemingly unbridgeable states of mind. The insights developed here seem to be at the very core of Bion's clinical work. Bion asserted that, in order to approach the patient's logic, the analyst had to penetrate or transcend the caesura of their own logic – or the logic of the conscious, finite, awake mind – and give their imagination an airing so as to encounter a different logic, seemingly irrational, or perhaps 'anti-rational'.

Referring to this concept, Bergstein asserts that this paper also underscores the significance of working in the immediacy of the here and now with the prospect of expanding one's capacity to tolerate contact with reality in transit, in the unfolding present. The discourse of "caesura" clearly implies a discourse on method, intended by Bion to give theoretical tools to the analyst in order to help him or her to remain open to emotional turbulence.

I will now refer to Chapter 10, "Transformations", written by João Carlos Braga. Bion began the study of the transitions between the elements of psychoanalysis by means of PS-D, C–c, and selected fact in *Learning from Experience* (1962b) and *Elements of Psychoanalysis* (1963). He continued in *Transformations* (1965), studying these transitions in more detail and making use of the geometrical theory of transformations. His aim was to develop better instruments for observation. For Bion, the theory of transformations is a theory of psychoanalytic observation.

Despite the inherent challenges in comprehending and extracting the full benefits from Bion's seminal work, for Braga, *Transformations* (1965) stands as an invaluable repository of Bion's dedicated efforts to advance our understanding of the workings of the human mind. Braga lucidly and astutely plunges into the text, considering that this book is notably replete with profound observations and practical proposals relevant to clinical practice. Bion reformulates the concept of conscious and unconscious as finite and infinite; suggests that the concept of transformation marks a paradigm shift in regard to the Freudian idea of distortion; offers a theory of temporality through the psychoanalytic account of the dialectic between being and being-there; and, finally, with the conceptual triad of O, invariance, and transformation, sketches the outline of a complex theory of knowledge. Detailed clinical examples are also present in Braga's contribution, as he searches to find a clinical usefulness even for abstract ideas. I have always greatly appreciated Braga's unique ability to address difficult issues with great lucidity and a clear and communicative writing style, and, in the discussion in this chapter, these qualities shine to the fullest.

By the end of *Transformations*, Bion reaches the insight that one cannot know the origin, O, of what is transformed. This provides the basis for a shift in which he changes his focus from the representations of experiences (K) to the unknowable reality itself that is behind these representations (O) and to the transformations that happen at this level (transformations in O). As pointed out by Vermote (2019), along with the algebraic notion of infinity, Bion comes to rely on Platonic forms and the Kantian thing-in-itself, finally borrowing expressions from the mystics who, throughout the ages, had also been confronted with the task of apprehending and conveying unknowable, ineffable experience.

Bion adumbrated the concept of 'the language of achievement' in *Learning from Experience* (1962b), but he developed it more fully in *Attention and Interpretation* (1970). He borrowed the term 'achievement' from Keats, along with 'negative capability' – which is achievement's obligatory counterpart – and applied the concept of language of achievement to the analyst's interaction with the patient. Ordinary language, which is sensuously derived and which Bion calls the language of substitution, is based upon representations of objects – that is, substitutive symbols derived from the sense organs.

The title of Afsaneh Kiany Alisobhani's Chapter 11, "Negative Capability: Navigating the Paradox in the Language of Achievement and the Language of Substitution", captures the essence of Bion's contribution. She suggests that the term 'language of achievement' belongs to a pre-symbolic lexicon approaching the truth of emotional experience in analysis. Only interpretations informed by such emotional experiences are transformative. Their truthfulness permeates the domain of time and space. For Bion, the language of achievement is the primal language of emotions (Bion 1970), and, for Grotstein (2007), the language of achievement is the paradoxical, apophatic language of becoming.

The importance of transformation in hallucinosis and language of substitution in approximating the language of achievement is illustrated through a clinical example showing the clinical implications of the notions of language of achievement (negative capability – as a primary tool in the endeavour of approaching unknowable ultimate reality). In this vignette, we see Alisobhani operationalizing the communicative aspect of projective identification and the view that the patient comes to analysis seeking an object who can receive, hold, and help him or her transform the primitive distress that is overwhelming him or her and is being projected into the analyst – that there is an urge in each of us to communicate emotional experience as a driving force in psychic growth and development.

With patience and security, Alisobhani, in her clinical example, suspended the distracting din of the language of substitution so as to keep herself open to the unconscious emotions that are spontaneously welling up from within herself as she fully experiences herself experiencing the full presence of the analysand – that is, experiencing 'becoming' O from within herself that is resonant with the patient's O. In doing this, it is here that the analyst is called upon to make his or her mind available; to be deeply receptive, willing to resonate with the patient and put an end to the war in the mind from which the patient may be suffering; to help the patient to rediscover the link between sensoriality and thoughts and bring him or her back to the original nest where he or she was born and from where he or she may grow and flourish.

Final Reflections

In closing, let me say that conveying all the riches that await the reader in this book can be challenging. Through eleven chapters, international authors offer expansions and extensions of contemporary and timeless themes. Another merit of the book is to show us the originality with which psychoanalysts from different geographical regions take ownership of the ideas discussed. The authors reveal to us the elements of continuity and discontinuity in Bion's work, sharing open conjectures to allow new developments to evolve. Every thought seems to engender knowledge and give birth to new hypotheses and theories that enter the torrent of their reflections and arrive transformed by communication; no idea is presented merely for contemplation: all are generously offered as an opportunity to think, change, and create.

It is inspiring that each of these readings leads to different ways of working and understanding our work and confirms that the transformational power of psychoanalysis lies in the possibility of sharing experiences with colleagues from all regions with respect, openness, amazement, and freedom.

I no longer want to detain the reader in the pleasure of the encounter and so I invite you to echo Bion's suggestion: "with certain books one does not 'read' them – one has to have an emotional experience of reading them".

References

Abel-Hirsch, N. (2023). *Bion: An Introduction*. Phoenix.
Bion, W.R. (1958). On arrogance. *International Journal of Psychoanalysis*, 39, 144–146.
Bion, W.R. (1962a). A theory of thinking. In *Second Thoughts*. Aronson.
Bion, W.R. (1962b). *Learning from Experience*. Basic Books.
Bion, W.R. (1963, 2014). Vol. 5. *Elements of Psycho-Analysis*. In The Complete Works of W.R. Bion. Routledge.

Bion, W.R. (1965, 2014). Vol. 5. *Transformations: Change from Learning to Growth*. In The Complete Works of W.R. Bion. Routledge.

Bion, W.R. (1967a, 2014). Vol. 6. *Notes on Memory and Desire*. In The Complete Works of W.R. Bion. Routledge.

Bion, W.R. (1967b, 2014). Vol. 6. *Second Thoughts: Selected Papers on Psycho-Analysis*. In The Complete Works of W.R. Bion. Routledge.

Bion, W.R. (1970, 2014). Vol. 6. *Attention and Interpretation: A Scientific Approach to Insight in Psycho-Analysis and Groups*. In The Complete Works of W.R. Bion. Routledge.

Bion, W.R. (1977a, 2014). Vol. 13. *A Memoir of the Future: Book 2*. In The Complete Works of W.R. Bion. Routledge.

Bion, W.R. (1977b). *Two Papers: 'The Grid' and 'Caesura'*. Imago.

Bion, W.R. (1979, 2014). Vol. 14. *A Memoir of the Future: Book 3*. In The Complete Works of W.R. Bion. Routledge.

Bion, W.R. (1980). *Bion in New York and São Paulo*. Clunie.

Bion, W.R. (1982, 2014). Vol. 1. *The Long Weekend 1897–1919: Part of a Life*. The Complete Works of W.R. Bion. Routledge.

Bion, W.R. (1985, 2014). Vol. 2. *My Sins Remembered: Another Part of a Life, The Other Side of Genius: Family Letters*. In The Complete Works of W.R. Bion. Routledge.

Bion, W.R. (1997, 2014). Vol. 3. *War Memoirs 1917–1919*. In The Complete Works of W.R. Bion. Routledge.

Bleandonu G, (1993). *Wilfred R. Bion: His Life and Works*. Free Association Books.

Brown, L. J. (2012). Bion's discovery of alpha function: Thinking under fire on the battlefield and in the consulting room. *International Journal of Psychoanalysis*, 93: 1191–1214.

Freud, S. (1911). Formulations on the two principles of mental functioning. *The Standard Edition of the Complete Psychological Works of Sigmund Freud*, Vol. 12, pp. 213–226. Hogarth.

Grotstein, J.S. (2007). *A Beam of Intense Darkness*. Karnac.

Harris Williams, M. (2010). *Bion's Dream: A Reading of the Autobiographies*. Routledge.

Smith, T. (2021). 'Half alive, half dead' boys: sexuality and censorship in Wilfred Bion's The Long Weekend. *Journal of Child Psychotherapy*.

Smith, T. (2023). *The Tiger Skin on the Bannister (and Other Stories): Internal Dialogues and Parallel Autobiographical Process in a Reading of Wilfred Bion's The Long Weekend*.

Vermote, R. (2019). *Reading Bion*. Karnac Books.

Bion Bibliography

Bion, W.R. (2014). The Complete Works of W.R. Bion. Edited by C. Mawson and F. Bion. Routledge.

Bion, W.R. (1982, 2014). Vol. 1. *The Long Weekend 1897–1919: Part of a Life*. In The Complete Works of W.R. Bion. Routledge.

Bion, W.R. (1985, 2014). Vol. 2. *My Sins Remembered: Another Part of a Life & The Other Side of Genius: Family Letters*. In The Complete Works of W.R. Bion. Routledge.

Bion, W.R. (1997, 2014). Vol. 3. *War Memoirs 1917–1919*. In The Complete Works of W.R. Bion. Routledge.

Bion, W.R. (2014). Vol. 4. The 'War of Nerves' (1940); On Groups (1943); The Leaderless Group Project (1946); Psychiatry at a Time of Crisis (1948); Group Methods of Treatment (1948); Language and the Schizophrenic (1955); Experiences in Groups and Other Papers (1961); Learning from Experience (1962). In The Complete Works of W.R. Bion. Routledge.

Bion, W.R. (2014). Vol. 5. Elements of Psycho-Analysis (1963); Taming Wild Thoughts (I): The Grid (1963); Transformations: Change from Learning to Growth (1965). In The Complete Works of W.R. Bion. Routledge.

Bion, W.R. (2014). Vol. 6. Memory and Desire (1965); Catastrophic Change (1966); Second Thoughts: Selected Papers on Psychoanalysis (1967); Notes on Memory and Desire (1967); Attention and Interpretation: A Scientific Approach to Insight in Psycho-Analysis and Groups (1970); Book Reviews (1966). In The Complete Works of W.R. Bion. Routledge.

Bion, W.R. (2014). Vol. 7. Brazilian Lectures: 1973 São Paulo Lectures; 1974 São Paulo Lectures; 1974 Rio de Janeiro Lectures. In The Complete Works of W.R. Bion. Routledge.

Bion, W.R. (2014). Vol. 8. Clinical Seminars: Brasilia 1975. Contributions to Panel Discussions: Brasilia, a New Experience (1975); São Paulo (1978). Bion in New York and São Paulo: New York (1977); São Paulo (Ten talks) (1978). In The Complete Works of W.R. Bion. Routledge.

Bion, W.R. (2014). Vol. 9. The Tavistock Seminars (June 1976–March 1979); The Italian Seminars (1977); A Paris Seminar (July 1978). In The Complete Works of W.R. Bion. Routledge.

Bion, W.R. (2014). Vol. 10. Two Papers: The Grid (1971); Caesura (1975). Four Discussions (1976). Four Papers: Emotional Turbulence (1976); On a Quotation from Freud (1976); Evidence (1976); Making the Best of a Bad Job (1979). Interview with Anthony Banet Jnr (1976). Taming Wild Thoughts (II): Untitled (1977). In The Complete Works of W.R. Bion. Routledge.

Bion, W.R. (2014). Vol. 11. Cogitations. Review of Cogitations, by André Green. In The Complete Works of W.R. Bion. Routledge.

Bion, W.R. (2014). Vol. 12. *A Memoir of the Future: Book 1*. In The Complete Works of W.R. Bion. Routledge.

Bion, W.R. (2014). Vol. 13. *A Memoir of the Future: Book 2*. In The Complete Works of W.R. Bion. Routledge.

Bion, W.R. (2014). Vol. 14. *A Memoir of the Future: Book 3* (with expanded key). In The Complete Works of W.R. Bion. Routledge.

Bion, W.R. (2014). Vol. 15. Unpublished papers: The Conception of Man (1961); Penetrating Silence (1976); New and Improved (1977); Further Cogitations (1968–1969). In The Complete Works of W.R. Bion. Routledge.

Bion, W.R. (2014). Vol. 16. *References General*. In The Complete Works of W.R. Bion. Routledge.

Chapter 1

Reading the Child and Adolescent Bion[1]

Tim Smith

This chapter is based on two previously published papers, '"Half alive, half dead" boys: Sexuality and censorship in Wilfred Bion's "The long weekend"' (Smith, 2021) and 'The tiger skin on the bannister (and other stories): Internal dialogues and parallel autobiographical process in a reading of Wilfred Bion's *The Long Weekend, 1897–1919: Part of a Life*' (Smith, 2023), published by Routledge.

Introduction

In recent research, I've been especially interested in the varied states of mind that Bion recalled in his autobiography about his childhood, adolescence and young adulthood, *The Long Weekend, 1897–1919: Part of a Life* (1982; see Smith, 2021, 2023). His life writing raises interesting questions for me about (1) masculinity and boys becoming men from a psychoanalytic perspective, (2) the forced separation of young British boys from their parents in the Edwardian era and, (3) the process of trauma on the lives of young men pre-World War I, especially in Britain. But, and as I researched (Smith, 2021), I think it also has something to say about the nature of adolescent states of mind in general – perhaps there is even a theory of adolescence to be found within it – as well as clues to the origins of some of Bion's great theories.

Bion's book, written when he was eighty years old, after all his theories had been published, is divided into three parts – 'India', 'England' and 'War' – and covers the first twenty-one years of his life. Born in Muttra, northwest India, he was sent to England at the young age of eight years old. Voyages such as these were a common occurrence for children from British families in what was known as the Raj at that time, although not without their emotional consequences. Excruciatingly, for Bion, it meant that he never saw his much-loved ayah again and, according to his second wife, Francesca Bion, he went without seeing his mother for the next three years (Bion, 1995, p. 91), although the timeline is much less clear in Bion's own text. My reading is that Bion's vague timeline conveys the feeling quality of the agonising waits he endured between his mother's visits to him at the school, and the way the

DOI: 10.4324/9781032661230-2

pain of his abandonment led him to feel overwhelmingly uncertain as to where she was in his mind. He remained at the school – Bishop's Stortford College in Hertfordshire – where bullying was rife and the staff were, at times, negligent in their responsibilities for looking after children, especially in the prep school, for the following ten years.

Upon finishing there, he enlisted as a soldier, successful only on the second attempt – and with help from his father, which he resented – to go and fight on the battlefields of France in World War I. The descriptions of his war-time experiences, including that he was the only member of his tank regiment to survive, are perhaps better known than those he suffered at his Hertfordshire boarding school. However, it is clear from the account of his schooldays – the section 'England', my focus in this chapter – that his psychic survival was something he grappled with well before the war. I especially centre my thoughts around the psychically disruptive early experiences and states of mind pertaining to sexuality and masculinity, from a psychoanalytic developmental point of view, that Bion describes he moved in and out of as a child and adolescent. I pay attention to the social context – that is, the emotional atmosphere – he grew up in and the impact this had on him. And, briefly, I describe a process of personal reverie that helped me make sense of the emotional content of Bion's descriptions of himself as a child and adolescent.

Some Comments on Autobiography and Reading an Autobiography

Autobiography, within the field of life writing, has inherent problems with individualism/subjectivity. On the one hand, it gets criticised for the many complexities associated with remembering and reconstructing, as an area too fraught to retain any relationship to objectivity. On the other hand, however, subjectivity – that is, 'how individuals construct meaning' (Harrison, 2009, p. xxxii) – is an inevitable and important aspect of our lives and in making sense of experiences. And, accounts with limited subjectivity, where the complexities of feelings and relationships are evaded, can only ever provide a limited picture.

A further complexity is that socio-political forces can contribute to resistances in exploring subjective terrains and, at times, therefore, in bringing non-dominant narratives into the wider public view. For example, within the survivor subgenre, usually written by adult survivors of childhood abuse and neglect, stories may not always be believed, and it can be seen how dominant socio-political forces may gang up to perpetuate the crime of a robbed childhood. I have argued (Smith, 2021; see also Douglas, 2010; Hodgkin & Radstone, 2003/2017; Walker, 2003/2017) that accusations that the autobiographical method is invalid as a reliable source of information are, perhaps, most likely to occur when there are perceived or actual dangers with authenticity. Indeed, imbalances of power that are prevalent when children in society suffer can begin to shift and even threaten socially accepted norms when the experiences of victims of childhood maltreatment are brought into public awareness. I think that child psychotherapists and child analysts, perhaps especially those who work in state-run institutions, are often acutely familiar with the stories of children who are felt to tell tales which, when listened to, often contain powerful emotional truths.

The term 'psychoanalytic autobiography' – and I think Bion's book is a great example – describes a special subgenre of autobiography interested in matters of truth and derived from processes of interior observation. (Harris Williams argues that psychoanalytic autobiography is, like psychoanalysis, another deeply powerful means of introducing the patient to themself [2012, p. 398]). My own view is that psychoanalytic autobiography can provide vital and valuable perspectives, what I have called 'routes to intimate truths' (Smith, 2021). While it has been criticised (see, especially, Ehrlich, 2017), I think *The Long Weekend* reliably takes the reader on a journey towards witnessing these intimate truths. It is the inside story of Bion's severely emotionally deprived and psychically disrupted development.

Bion sets out explicitly that he aims only to be 'relatively truthful' (1982, p. 9) in his account. He is aware that this is all he can be. Indeed, he notes the complexities of memory in his earlier writing output – see *Notes on Memory and Desire*, where he states that memory is 'always misleading as a record of fact' owing to the forces of unconscious mental life (1967, p. 205). The central aim in his book is to recall his inner states, and his depictions of his states of mind have the value of subjectivity. In *Transformations* (1965), Bion had understood as central to the transference process 'to understand the patient's view of the analyst's view of the patient' and how this can give a description of phantasy and the transference as key to psychoanalytic understanding.

The method I apply to reading Bion's book is similar to Holmes's 'reverie research' methodology for research interviews and reading psychoanalytic texts (Holmes, 2018a, 2018b). It allows for the use of my subjective responses to a text, including more disturbing associations and memories, by exercising 'alpha function' (Bion, 1962). And, I also draw on contemporary psychoanalytic conceptions of the adolescent process and a limited number of relevant socio-historical texts, and other autobiographical writing, to add a further perspective to the one Bion chose to provide.

Sexuality

Bion is not especially known for writing about sexuality in his extensive theoretical contributions to psychoanalysis. However, one of the pervasive states of mind I encounter in his text is a heavily repressed sexuality. And, as well as the difficulties he faces from the inside, he chooses to emphasise the destructive moral and religious attitudes of the day that contributed to this repression.

The Problem of Sex

His sexual development was frightening to him in the starkest of senses; he describes in no uncertain terms how sex was a 'PROBLEM' (1982, p. 106, his emphasis). And, the chapters in which he writes about this (especially Chapters 4 and 5, pp. 55–65, detailing his masturbatory behaviour in the prep school; Chapters 11 and 12, pp. 87–93, and Chapter 15, pp. 106–108, describing his pubertal development in the main school) are, to read, some of the most enigmatic and perplexing in the entire section 'England'. While sex is put left, right, front and centre in these chapters, at the same time it is written about with a peculiar kind of censorship. For example, Bion writes: 'One [school] house in particular was notorious for ... what?' (p. 92). I read his censoring as being bound up with both boarding school culture and the child and adolescent Bion's own struggles – a Bion who was, arguably, himself a neglected child. I am referring to the kind of 'double deprivation' (Williams, 1997/2002) that occurs on the inside in response to heavily deprived external circumstances. (I wish to note that I do not think his background of prosperity and privilege made him immune to experiencing serious deprivations.)

Bion also interjects his account of intensely painful experiences using an authorial 'performativity', adopting a rather joking, yet elusive, writing style. There are various interpretations that could be made as to why. Perhaps to provide some light relief to the simply staggering misery and suffering described in his autobiographical drama; or perhaps to portray, with the use of omission ('for ... what?') how as a child he had to split off any conscious or physical awareness of some events (see also Waddell, 2013, p. 17)? Often, Bion *pretends* to adhere to the stringent moral and religious attitudes towards sex of the day. For example, naming something such as masturbation, despite its inevitability in adolescence – not least at a segregated public boys' school – was considered a dangerous venture, for reasons I will come to.

Furthermore, the lack of creativity at the school, where there was an 'absolute hatred and loathing of sexuality' (Bion, 1982, p. 87), is conveyed vividly by Bion with his descriptions of boys who are 'half alive' and 'half dead' (p. 116). He states that the destructive emotional atmosphere effectively sought to 'dam back the noxious matter til it stank' and 'buried' the growth of his personality (p. 108). He describes how, as a child and adolescent boy, he was in need of serious help with the above matters. However, within the context of a 'web of undirected menace' (pp. 59, 107), none of his schoolmasters were able to provide him with this support. Teaching about sex and relationships was not 'in the prospectus' (p. 93). Only problematic and brutalising solutions to the problem of sex in segregated boarding schools existed: notably the fagging system, a deeply entrenched structure for managing the domestic lives of boys, as well as 'substitution[s]' (p. 108), primarily intensely competitive sports. I think he refused to call these sublimations, not yet a Freudian term, knowing the reader would think this, as he wished to emphasise the harmful impact of the system that was not for creative purposes. There was also religion, which Harris Williams notes seemed to function as a kind of 'regulator of sexual desires' (2010, p. 11). At these schools, pubescent boys essentially had to find their own way through the physical and emotional upheavals associated with their development, amid the control and surveillance mechanisms of their schoolmasters who created networks of 'honourable spying' (Bion, 1982, p. 90).

The impact of all this on Bion was long-standing and arresting. He considered himself sexually immature and continued feeling disturbed as a young adult. He wrote in the second part of his autobiography, *All My Sins Remembered: Another Part of a Life* (Bion, 1985), how, shortly after the war, he briefly fell in love with a young woman and felt incredibly rejected when she lavished her attentions on someone else. One day, and by coincidence, when he saw her together with her new lover at the beach, he felt humiliated and had violent fantasies about shooting them and causing the couple permanent damage (pp. 29–30).

There is also the mention of an allegation made against Bion by a student's mother when he returned to teach at the school in his twenties, that he made advances towards her son – unsubstantiated claims (Vermote, 2019), although he left the school at this point and, it seems, did not access legal advice. Is it possible that, in his disturbed state of mind, having returned from the war and following graduating from Oxford University, given what we know about his disrupted childhood development, he got entangled in something here?

Early Context

Adolescence is a 'secondary individuation' (Blos, 1967) with its roots in infancy, and Bion does include some account of his infantile sexuality in the section 'India'. I think he provides the clues in that section as to his later (over)reliance on masturbation via descriptions of the context of his early home life. He had been an inquisitive young child with a tendency to be cruel to his younger sister, whom he disliked, and his parents lacked emotional resources. It seems they'd found his character and his differences to them difficult to tolerate. His mother could be unpredictable: in one moment 'warm safe and comfortable', but the next 'cold and frightening' (Bion, 1982, p. 13) – it is probable she was depressed. (In *All My Sins Remembered* he describes his parents as 'completely cracked'.) His father, meanwhile, sometimes became frustrated with him and was prone to 'burst' into fits of rage that involved turning Bion upside down to give him a 'good beating' (p. 15).

Bion writes that he first discovered 'the pleasure of masturbation by lying on my stomach on the floor and wriggling' (p. 30), something his sister could make nothing of. He was still a young child and recalls his masturbatory behaviour drew a peculiarly confused and confusing response from his parents, whose expressions were 'frozen' when they noticed, and yet, bizarrely, they still picked him up and kissed him without saying a word. Subsequently, Bion describes feeling guilty, as if 'bits of the Bible' were stuck to him 'like fluff' that he couldn't get off himself (p. 30). However, he also recalls giggling when his parents found him out, conveying considerable ambivalence (p. 31). It was, after all, something he discovered he could do without them, exciting, self-soothing, and presumably a way of removing himself from the emotional atmosphere of bleak family discord in which he was growing up.

So, what Bion details is, at one level, nothing more than any boy's inevitable discovery. However, what seemed to have been problematic was his parents' response, which occurred in the context of his feelings of significant despair. No understanding and no helpful prohibitions were supplied; only what Bion later described as a 'moral foam', which his father used to 'extinguish' him with (p. 127). They were perhaps entangled, like other parents at that time, in the same web of undirected menace that was at work in the school system: an evangelical, moral and religious atmosphere widespread throughout the British Empire. Therefore, they could not voice or provide appropriate help, let alone think to understand, in the matter of their young son's masturbatory behaviour. Bion emphasises that he grew up in 'pre-Freudian days' (p. 106) – that is, before the acknowledgement of infantile sexuality and the proliferation of Freud's ideas.

One thought I have is that his parents' silence likely contributed to his own emerging belief that he did not need any help – an incredibly painful thread to his writing, but an omnipotent denial of reality and a reliance on what he went on to call the 'Lie' (pp. 44–45; capital letter inserted by author) once he reached the prep school. I see the 'Lie' as referring to an internal, gang-like constellation that came into being with the events of his traumatic arrival at the prep school and closed its grip on him over the course of his schooldays, resulting in the disastrous situation whereby he could not make meaningful contact with people and rejected almost all dependencies. This 'Lie' took him away from one of the realities of life – his ordinary need for help (Stokoe, 2021, p. 3, after Money-Kyrle, 1971, p. 103). Loneliness causes the 'Lie'. Small wonder that Bion's life's work, once he realised these things, was to point out the necessity for 'container–contained' (Bion, 1970) relationships.

Latency and Early Adolescence

Bion was separated from his ayah and homeland, both of whom he was very fond of, and everything familiar to him when he made the journey from India to England aged eight. He then felt utterly abandoned when his mother left him at the prep school. His description of watching her hat go bobbing up and down and away from him over the school hedge (1982, p. 43) tugs on the heart strings. And, subsequently, he was severely bullied, emotionally and physically, not helped by being both the smallest as well as the youngest child when he arrived at the prep school, reminding his peers of their absent mothers, as Waddell also notes (2018, p. 111). In his emotionally vulnerable, newly arrived state, he was a convenient recipient for their unbearable feelings of being abandoned, which, in fact, they all shared.

Oedipal issues also dominate the text. I think Bion implies that his desire for his mother within this painful set of circumstances only led to fears of further loss, when the headmaster Hirst, who can be viewed as a paternal substitute, threatened him with expulsion for masturbating. He was terrified when Hirst noticed and told him, 'Don't do that Wilfred [...] or you will have to be sent away' (p. 50). This time there were prohibitions set, although, agonisingly, still no understanding afforded to him (p. 50). He recalls how the other boys stared 'in stony innocence' (p. 50), ostracising him, as if none of them were at it in private, leaving him to feel increasingly anxious.

Curiously, he adopts the term 'wiggling' (p. 50) in the text as code for masturbation, at the point he arrives at the prep school and onwards. His furious activity spilled out quickly from the less than private location of his dormitory bed to the quite public forum of the classroom, where it seems his inhibitions almost entirely disappeared, such was his immersion in the activity. However, Bion's choice of word – 'wiggling' – emphasises the infantile aspect, although he jokes that his masturbation 'could hardly have been more anonymous than the Indian bear's progress through the forest' (p. 50). The repeated use of jokes about his painful circumstances, both inner and outer, seems to have been one way he had of holding himself together as a child. I suspect it may also have been a helpful way for the eighty-year-old Bion to look back at his acutely painful childhood in order to write about it.

One day, Hirst lectured the students following a serious incident between two boys that had led, on this occasion, to an older child being removed from the school (pp. 57–58). Hirst implored the boys to speak up if they ever became aware of peers 'poisoning the mind' of others. Bion became confused by this expression and thought, concretely, that a boy's food had been poisoned, which had resulted in their death. Scared, he asked the boy who was sitting next to him who it was that had died, only to be told 'I'll tell you later' (p. 58). Realising he had misunderstood something, he concluded that the boy must have been sent away for wiggling. It was not until Bion moved up to the main school that he worked out that the older boy had been expelled for engaging in sexual activity with a younger child (p. 90) – 'for ... what?' (p. 92).

Increasingly terrified about the prospects of expulsion, Bion resolved to give up wiggling forever but found that this was not that easy(!) as 'it did not and would not give me up' (p. 58) – a reference to the onset of puberty, outside his control. He writes,

> I had no luck at all. I might resolve to have nothing to do with wiggling, but wiggling did not return the compliment. What was more I felt so much better – even so morally better – after wiggling, and far more able to withstand temptation. I almost entered into lavish contracts with the

Almighty to leave my 'widdler' alone. I sometimes wondered if Saint Paul was speaking metaphorically about his 'thorn in the flesh'; my 'widdler' was permanently stuck into my flesh. (p. 60)

His pubescent development, with its 'thorn in the flesh' (p. 60) erections, brought about a further source of pain for him. I think Bion intends his masturbatory behaviour be understood as a further defensive structure, holding him together in the absence of any support, a source of warmth in the cold prep school climate, where he worried 'boys died off like flies' (p. 47) and little else was available to him. He conveys feeling desperately anxious, as if there really was no place for him in anyone's mind, and as if he deserved his terrible suffering. He writes that, by the time he moved up to the main school, 'I had reduced my sexual life to perfunctory prayers of the "Oh God, save me from self-abuse" type' (p. 92). At the same time, masturbation was 'the only redeeming thing', making him feel, almost instantly, 'so much better' (p. 60), although it contributed to increasing layers of guilt. Nearing the end of the prep school, by now a physically developing boy, Bion had developed an exceptionally harsh, self-deprecating attitude, calling himself 'a bad boy, a dirty little wiggling horrid boy' (p. 59). He was clearly very depressed.

Socio-historical Atmosphere

Ordinary sexual explorations between boys in segregated public boarding schools were and remain common and inevitable. Segregation from girls and women is an important matter in the book, as repression can also be linked to the all-male context. This was something that had further ramifications for adolescent boys of Bion's time, as well as the women who looked after them, who went to go and fight in the war. It is a running theme in 'England' with the boys sequestered from their mothers from a young age: the headmaster Hirst's wife was rumoured to have been away at an asylum (in Bion's mind for masturbating too much), while other schoolmasters, such as the classics teacher Colman, appeared not to have sexual relationships. There was problem: what to do with sex in these environments?

The poet and novelist Graves, a contemporary of Bion who went to Charterhouse boarding school, wrote in his autobiography *Goodbye to All That* that sexual intimacy was 'almost always between boys of the same age who were not in love, and used each other as convenient sex-instruments' and 'the atmosphere was always heavy with romance of a conventional early-Victorian type' (Graves, 2000, p. 39). Graves, like Bion, was terribly unhappy at public school, calling it a 'fundamental evil' (p. 36), and wrote to his father at one point desperately requesting his withdrawal. Along similar lines, the biographer and social historian Gathorne-Hardy notes in his excellent book *The Old School Tie: The Phenomenon of the English Public School* how, for some, given how miserable things felt, romantic sexual encounters were perhaps 'the only happy moments' that boys knew (1977, p. 161). Sadly, within these environments, there also existed all too frequent incidents of serious abuses of younger boys by older boys and masters. Graves alludes to this, writing that the atmosphere was 'complicated by cynicism and foulness' (2000, p. 39); and Gathorne-Hardy is explicit in his historical account of the activities that went on, how the fear of sexual advances from older boys was in fact so great that it often led to attempts to keep the age groups distinctly apart (1977, p. 166).

Indeed, prior to the Edwardian era, the Victorian authorities had become increasingly concerned by reports of neglect, extreme cruelty and physical and sexual abuse between boys and their schoolmasters, adding to the impoverished conditions in public schools of the age. This became something of a national scandal, and the Public Schools Act, 1868, was brought in to attempt reform and regulate seven of the leading English schools, although difficulties remained widespread. In dire circumstances such as these, it was felt that young boys needed to know what masturbation and sex were, in an attempt to protect them. At the same time, bafflingly, it was feared that having grown-ups talking to them about these matters would only increase the prevalence of sexual activity, as well as the consequences the Victorians attached to it in fantasy, infused with religious interpretations. (In the Old Testament story, Onan was a man who refused to marry his widowed sister-in-law and instead 'spilled his seed' [semen] on the ground, for which he was killed by God in punishment. It is also a story that does not allow any space for the emotional responses to a tragic family drama, where procreation is seen as the sole demand.) Hence the widely canvassed myth at the time that masturbation led to insanity and an early death.

One attempt, then popular but now heavily berated, at teaching children about the perceived dangers of masturbation was led by Dean Frederic Farrar, who wrote several children's morality tales. The most notorious of Farrar's books, *Eric, or Little by Little* (1858), is a text Bion references several times in *The Long Weekend*. The book epitomises the cultural panic of the 1850s and 1860s, although its ripple effects were still widely felt in the Edwardian era when Bion was at school. The character of Eric is, like Bion, a boy from a British family in the Raj sent to boarding school in England. Despite being descended from nobility, he becomes slowly demoralised by being punished unfairly for wrongdoings. He is also bullied (something Farrar is unable to attend to) before starting to go off the rails – drinking, smoking, cheating and then running off to sea with pirates. Finally, at the end of the tale, he sees the error of his ways and repents, just before his early and tragic death. However, 'the real core of the book's sermon' (Roberts, 2013) is the danger of that unnameable activity: masturbation. Farrar writes,

> May every schoolboy who reads this page be warned by the waving of their wasted hands, from that burning marle of passion where they found nothing but shame and ruin, polluted affections, and an early grave. (1858)

Several famous authors, including Kipling in his book *Stalky & Co.* (1899), which takes a more worldly view of adolescent boys growing up in British boarding schools, ridicule *Eric*, and the book's lasting impact has been described as 'an immortality of derision' (Richards, 1988), although Bion writes, 'we did not use the term "masturbation", and were too "refined" to use others available to "rough boys"' (1982, p. 106) – the only time in the section 'England' that he names the activity face on.

Early to Mid-Adolescence

Bion's references to homosexuality oscillate with descriptions of love for mothers and an awakening desire for girls. He had two friends with whose families he stayed during school holidays – Heaton Rhodes and John Dudley Hamilton. It is perhaps not so curious, given the above context, that Bion describes feeling nothing when one night, unexpectedly, as he was lying in bed with his pyjamas on, his friend Dudley 'suddenly discarded the towel he had round his waist and jumped astride me as if challenging me to wrestle' (p. 87). Dudley's impromptu abandonment of his towel represents the emotional quality of the abrupt and unpredictable physical changes precursory to the boys' pubertal developments in the main school. The not-quite, quasi-wrestling is communicative of the questions all pubescent children have about how sexually developed beings get together and the capabilities they are about to acquire.

However, Bion's response conveys a stifling of sexuality on the inside as well. Dudley, having got on top of him, said to Bion, 'Now how do you feel?' (p. 87). Bion recalls, 'I felt nothing physically; mentally a sense of boredom and anti-climax, which soon communicated itself to Dudley who, after a few futile attempts to provoke a struggle, got off' (p. 87). When relaying the event to his first analyst, and I assume he means Mr FIP, not Rickman, Bion was convinced that they neither believed he had felt 'nothing', nor understood 'the horrible and painful nature of frustration, its powerful contribution, with fear and guilt, to an absolute loathing of sexuality in any shape or form' (p. 87). He seems to describe an internal state where sexuality and creativity were suffocated, a type of 'psychic retreat' (Steiner, 1993) manifesting as a persistent 'absence of passion' (Brady, 2017, p. 55) and adhered to as a way of dealing with the onset of sexuality and its developmental turbulence. Tragically, Bion goes on to recall how, as he and Dudley began to duel and wrestle in other forms, their friendship was lost, one of the few he had. He writes, 'the only overt and unmistakable emotional experience was when futility flared into mutual dislike, or more correctly, hate' (1982, pp. 87–88).

However, his stays with his two friends' families did provide him some much-needed respite from his miserable experiences at the school. Their mothers, Mrs Rhodes and especially Mrs Hamilton, were generally warm and loving – important to him as substitutes for his own mother and ayah whom he had lost early on. Internally, they were also renewed Oedipal figures with whom he was in love in early adolescence, and – also driven by the advancement of puberty – there were glimpses of a revival of his more passionate desires. One school holiday, spent at the Rhodes's farm, Bion took a shine to Heaton's sister, Kathleen – a 'pretty girl, tall and slender', who 'spoke straight' (p. 88). His feelings seem to stem from a genuine desire to connect with someone – a rare occurrence in his youth, given his tendency to reject relationships. He recalls being attracted to her 'fiery tempered' passion (p. 88), being able to see the truth in things and speak out against the established norms of the time, which she did despite it provoking her parents. Sadly, during his schooldays, Bion could not respond in a lively way to Kathleen's qualities, and he felt critical of himself for lacking the nerve to relate to her.

Reflections on Bion's Limited Acquisition of Masculine Identifications

Paternal Substitutes

Figlio argues that true identifications, that are not mere imitations, recognise reality and free boys to relate more generously and lovingly to women as they develop (2000, p. 120), and that identifications are important as boys need to find ways to relate to men other than as rivals, whereas imitations repudiate reality and are essentially narcissistic (p. 120). I want to spend a bit of time focussing my thoughts on the exceptionally limited availability of helpful masculine constructs present for Bion, as illustrated in his descriptions of the men who surrounded him at his boarding school – the likes of the teachers and his friends' fathers – and to reflect on his limited ability (although one can see some of this) to acquire masculine identifications.

Tellingly, Bion's own father barely receives a mention in the section 'England'. However, as a young child growing up in India, his father, a noted 'Big Game' shot (Bion, 1982, p. 21), is recalled as being prone to fits of rage and unable to sustain much patience with him. He (Bion's father) espoused, and was bound up with, colonial ideals of masculinity (a 'hypermasculinity'), epitomised in the event of the tiger hunt, which left Bion feeling scared at night that he would become the hunted himself, prey to the female tiger whose mate his father had shot (pp. 21–24).

With Hirst, the headmaster, who he describes frequently in this section, Bion seems to have had difficulty piecing together the man's complex character, which is made up of many different, unintegrated, parts. He conveys Hirst's varied qualities in his text: his dogged persistence at maintaining his composure and work function in a class with, at times, unruly adolescent boys, which they continually attempted to resist (pp. 94–95); his blind spots and ensuing neglectfulness; but also, his gentler side that captured the boys' curiosities and made them rather fond of him, given too their strong wishes to find some good identifications for themselves (pp. 55–56). Bion calls Hirst, poetically, 'my loved, unhappy, ghost-haunted failure' (1982, p. 116). I suggest a melancholy imitation (and I think also a melancholic internalisation and identification) rather than a healthy identification became established for Bion with Hirst. I also think the boys' denigration of their headmaster might have been, in part, an attempt to protect the more idealised versions of their mothers that they held (from whom they were separated).

A Personal Reverie or 'Parallel Autobiographical Process'

I referred earlier to the 'reverie research' methodology that I took as an approach to my reading of Bion's text. I knew that my own interest in Bion had something to do with my Indian paternal grandfather before I commenced my research. However, it was not until early in my work that I remembered my father once told me how he [my father] had attended a boarding school for delicate children where a haemophiliac boy in his dormitory had died. First, it took me by surprise to recall a familial link to boarding school culture, as it seemed removed from my own experiences at a day school. Second, I thought the similarity that my father's unprocessed experiences had to Bion's own painful circumstances was uncanny – Bion had been devastated when his unfortunate friend Freddie Sexton died from an acute bout of appendicitis. You will understand why I do not go into the ways I now imagine my father may have responded to his own painful event, other than to say that I think it is likely he latched on to some unhelpful masculine ideals that, it seems, were still prevalent in his own school half a century on from Bion's schooldays.

Later, I began to think further about my grandfather. I do not remember him, only some anecdotes from family members I grew up with. He died when I was an infant. I do know that, in his twenties, around the time of Partition, when the British Raj ended, he made the journey from India to Europe where he married my Dutch grandmother before settling in England. Unsure what to make of this connection, I then found myself, towards the end of my project, feeling distinctly unsettled by the cover of Bill Schwarz's book *Memories of Empire* (2011). The cover photo depicts a young, white British couple in the Raj posing in a jungle clearing behind a Bengal tiger. I noticed I made associations to a domestic cat – a creature that I love – before I realised the animal in the photograph had been hunted and was dead. Chillingly, I was looking at their kill laid out in front of them.

The following morning, I recalled the Indian tiger skin that had been draped, distinctly casually, over the bannister of my grandmother's staircase during my childhood. She kept it there long after my grandfather's death. The memory enabled me to connect with the way colonial constructs of masculinity had infiltrated my own domestic space, post-memory, in a silently destructive way while I was growing up. (The tiger skin was not something openly talked about, although my father's second wife sometimes expressed understandable discomfort about it.) It then made sense to me why I was interested to undertake an exploration of constructs of masculinity and masculine identifications as part of my analysis project. At the same time, this reflexive event helped me begin to consider the 'social memories' (Beiner, 2007) woven into Bion's recollections. (Beiner favours the term 'social memory' over 'collective memory', given what he sees as the non-reflexive use of the adjective 'collective' in many studies on memory, which he sees as allowing dominant narratives to hold sway.)

Increasingly aware of the devastating impact of imperialism in generating and sustaining the destructive macho attitudes of Bion's time, contained in his book, I began to notice more how he seems to use the characters of his friend Heaton Rhodes's father, Mr. Rhodes (see, especially, Bion, 1982, pp. 70–73), and the rather calcified headmaster of a neighbouring school, Thompson (pp. 116–117), to convey the infiltration of colonial ideals into his own domestic space. I noticed how, painfully, Bion internalised these ideals, and, by the end of his schooldays, his view of himself was as 'soft' and 'feminine' (p. 116) in the most disparaging, self-abasing sense – this in spite of growing into a young man with conventionally masculine skills, such as athletic prowess. (Although he was the youngest and smallest child when he arrived at the school, he grew into a fine rugby player, swimmer and runner in his adolescent years.)

Counterpoint

Briefly, it's important to mention that Bion was also interested in the Classics teacher Colman, who seemed a male figure able to offer him an opportunity to identify in a helpful way (and with whom he developed a more nurturing relationship), despite Colman having his own struggles (he was prone to crippling headaches that would send him 'dazed and almost reeling' out of the class [Bion, 1982, p. 115]). He is also alluded to as a pacifist. Crucially, Colman was able to help Bion catch sight of his rivalrousness with the other boys and not collude with it. He was also interested in thought and in mapping things out (pp. 111–115), a vital counterpoint to the false ideals of masculinity that infiltrated Bion's more general experiences. His Classics teacher seemed to have been an important prototype for Bion in later life, when his circumstances were more conducive to enable him to move on and learn from experience. Bion writes of Colman: 'though it was many years later before I had an idea of the extent of his benevolence, I could feel and be sustained by it' (p. 115). It feels especially tragic that Bion recalls viewing these more helpful experiences, at the time they occurred, as something of a luxury in his final years at the school, in the lead-up to going to fight on the battlefields of France in the war.

Concluding Remarks

The essence of *The Long Weekend* is, I think, a quite remarkable attempt to convey states of mind, recalled as near and as stripped-back as Bion could get to how they were, only possible given his lifetime's work devoted, but also being helped, to understand himself and others. The descriptions of his child and adolescent years, while comprising only a small section of the book, have distinct value. He describes sexual states of mind and masculine ideals/constructs during his child and adolescent years that did not propagate his creativity but caused him further pain, exacerbated feelings of abandonment, and found limited resolution. Bion presents himself as a passionate, yet strikingly repressed, adolescent, which led to personal limitations with sexuality (and possibly, too, contributing to the absence of the theme of sexuality in much of his writing). The impact of anxiety and deprivation on his inner life left him feeling only 'half alive' and also, in the most agonising of ways, 'half dead' (Bion, 1982, p. 116).

I think it is remarkable that, despite Bion's severely emotionally impoverished circumstances, there was some rekindling of his early infantile passions during his adolescence, seemingly enabled by the warmth and generosity of his friends' mothers, but also the capacity he had to observe the truth in things. (His capacity to observe, I think, also served to hold him together in a less defensive way – perhaps more 'endoskeleton' [Bion, 1982] than he gives himself credit for.) While fulfilling relationships did not really get going, the likes of his teacher Colman and friend's sister Kathy did provide him with important prototypes for more creative forms of relating, invaluable to him in later life (as Harris Williams [2010] also notes).

It was not only Bion who was frightened of his development; the culture and age feared it too – currents that still run very deep in our society today, including in the treatment of children. Bion was also a child of his time. The British Empire not only colonised the minds as well as the bodies of the colonised person, with devastating impacts (see especially Nandy, 1983, p. xi, and Treacher, 2007), but had a deeply damaging impact on the minds of the colonisers' children this way. However, perhaps the emphasis on the socio-historic atmosphere he grew up in, which contributed to stifling the growth of his personality (1982, p. 108), also attests to how we each can blame our propensity to repression and denial on the context around us, rather than on forces within us and ourselves. Bion's book still leaves us with much food for thought this way. The adolescent sexual states of mind Bion describes are still the kind that provoke much anxiety, disturbance and cause for concern in the public sphere, in the consulting room and in our workplaces today, but also, invariably – although less widely acknowledged – privately within oneself.

Dr Tim Smith is a child and adolescent psychotherapist and member of the Association of Child and Adolescent Psychotherapists in the UK. He works for the National Health Service and in private practice in East London.

Note

1 An earlier version of this paper was given at the Bion Seminars, Part II, organised by the Antonio Santamaria Foundation on 29 January 2023.

References

Beiner, G. (2007). *Remembering the Year of the French: Irish Folk History and Social Memory.* University of Wisconsin Press.

Bion, F. (1995, 2014). Vol. 15. *The Days of Our Years* (pp. 91–111). In The Complete Works of W.R. Bion. Routledge.

Bion, W.R. (1962, 2014). Vol. 4. *Learning from Experience* (pp. 247–365). In The Complete Works of W.R. Bion. Routledge.

Bion, W.R. (1965, 2014). Vol. 5. *Transformations* (pp. 115–280). In The Complete Works of W.R. Bion. Routledge.

Bion, W.R. (1967, 2014). Vol. 6. *Notes on Memory and Desire* (pp. 203–210). In The Complete Works of W.R. Bion. Routledge.

Bion, W.R. (1970, 2014). Vol. 6. *Attention and Interpretation: A Scientific Approach to Insight in Psychoanalysis and Groups* (pp. 211–330). In The Complete Works of W.R. Bion. Routledge.

Bion, W.R. (1982, 2014). Vol. 1. *The Long Weekend 1897–1919: Part of a Life* (pp. 1–318). In The Complete Works of W.R. Bion. Routledge.

Bion, W.R. (1985, 2014). Vol. 2. *All My Sins Remembered: Another Part of a Life and the Other Side of Genius: Family Letters* (pp. 1–265). In The Complete Works of W.R. Bion. Routledge.

Blos, P. (1967). The second individuation process of adolescence. *The Psychoanalytic Study of the Child*, 22(1), 162–186. doi:10.1080/00797308.1967.11822595

Brady, M. (2017). 'Sleeping beauties': Succession problems of adolescence. *Journal of Child Psychotherapy*, 43(1), 55–64. doi:10.1080/0075417X.2017.1283850

Douglas, K. (2010). *Contesting Childhood: Autobiography, Trauma and Memory.* Rutgers University Press.

Ehrlich, R. (2017). Bion's agony in *The Long Week-End. Journal of the American Psychoanalytic Association*, 65(4), 639–664.

Farrar, F. (1858). *Eric or, Little by Little.* Adam & Charles Black.

Figlio, K. (2000). *Psychoanalysis, Science and Masculinity.* Whurr.

Gathorne-Hardy, J. (1977). *The Old School Tie: The Phenomenon of the English Public School.* Viking Press.

Graves, R. (2000). *Goodbye to All That.* Penguin Classics. (Original work published 1929)

Harris Williams, M. (2010). *Bion's Dream: A Reading of the Autobiographies.* Routledge.

Harris Williams, M. (2012). On psychoanalytic autobiography. *Psychodynamic Practice*, 18(4), 397–412. doi:10.1080/14753634.2012.719737

Harrison, B. (2009). Editor's introduction: Researching lives and the lived experience. In B. Harrison (Ed.), *Life Story Research* (Vol. 1, pp. xxiii–xlviii). Sage.

Hodgkin, K., & Radstone, S. (2003/2017). Introduction: Contested pasts. In K. Hodgkin & S. Radstone (Eds.), *Memory, History, Nation: Contested Pasts (Memory & Narrative)* (pp. 1–22). Routledge.

Holmes, J. (2018a). Anorexia and the Trojan Horse: A reflexive review of written psychoanalytic encounters with anorexic patients. *Journal of Child Psychotherapy*, 45(1), 71–86. doi:10.1080/0075417X.2019.1617766

Holmes, J. (2018b). *A Practical Psychoanalytic Guide to Reflexive Research: The Reverie Research Method*. Routledge.

Kipling, R. (1899). *Stalky & Co*. Macmillan.

Money-Kyrle, R. (1971). The aim of psychoanalysis. *International Journal of Psychoanalysis*, 52(1) , 103–106. www.pep-web.org/document.php?id=ijp.052.0103a

Nandy, A. (1983). *The Intimate Enemy: Loss and Recovery of Self under Colonialism*. Oxford University Press.

Richards, J. (1988). *Happiest Days: The Public Schools in English Fiction*. Manchester University Press.

Roberts, A. (2013). Farrar's horcrux is wanking: 'Eric or, Little By Little' (1858) [online blog]. Retrieved January 1, 2020, from http://amechanicalart.blogspot.com/2013/10/farrars-horcruxis-.wanking-eric-or.html

Schwarz, Bill. (2011). *Memories of Empire: The White Man's World*. Oxford University Press.

Smith, T. (2021). 'Half alive, half dead' boys: Sexuality and censorship in Wilfred Bion's 'The long weekend'. *Journal of Child Psychotherapy*, 47(2), 296–312. doi:10.1080/0075417X.2021.1973538

Smith, T. (2023). The tiger skin on the bannister (and other stories): Internal dialogues and parallel autobiographical process in a reading of Wilfred Bion's *The Long Weekend, 1897–1919: Part of a Life*. *Life Writing*, 20(2), 421–434. doi:10.1080/14484528.2022.2046227

Steiner, J. (1993). *Psychic Retreats: Pathological Organizations in Psychotic, Neurotic and Borderline Patients*. Routledge.

Stokoe, P. (2021). *The Curiosity Drive: Our Need for Inquisitive Thinking*. Phoenix.

Treacher, A. (2007). Postcolonial subjectivity: Masculinity, shame, and memory. *Ethnic and Racial Studies*, 30(2), 281–299. doi:10.1080/01419870601143950

Vermote, R. (2019). *Reading Bion*. Routledge.

Waddell, M. (2013). Reflections on 'meaning' and 'meaningless' in post-Kleinian thought. In D. Bell & A . Novakovic (Eds.), *Living on the Border: Psychotic Processes in the Individual, the Couple and the Group* (pp. 11–27). The Tavistock Clinic Series. Routledge.

Waddell, M. (2018). *On Adolescence: Inside Stories*. The Tavistock Clinic Series. Routledge.

Walker, J. (2003/2017). The traumatic paradox: Autobiographical documentary and the psychology of memory. In K. Hodgkin & S. Radstone (Eds.), *Memory, History, Nation: Contested Pasts (Memory & Narrative)* (pp. 104–119). Routledge.

Williams, G. (1997/2002). Double deprivation. In *Internal Landscapes and Foreign Bodies: Eating Disorders and Other Pathologies* (pp. 33–50). Routledge.

Chapter 2

On Bion's "On Arrogance"

Peter Goldberg

Introduction

More than just a startlingly original paper, Bion's "On Arrogance" (1958) manages to incite the intense curiosity that the paper warns against. One is lured into wanting to know more – *What does he see in this peculiar troika of curiosity, stupidity, and arrogance? What does he mean by asserting that analysis is potentially complicit in realizing a psychical disaster?* – so that, by its end, this paper, as provocative as it is concise, may well have done what it warns about, adding fuel to the desire to know more of the truth of the deeper workings of the mind, a hunger that might take on the quality of arrogance and stupidity, as if we could actually know these truths.

Would it be an act of hubris, then, to attempt plumbing the meanings of this paper? But it is too late – having tasted this particular forbidden fruit of knowledge, we cannot now retract our curiosity without doing harm to the epistemophilic instincts. This is, after all, the dilemma that Bion reveals and forces us to confront in this paper – the dilemma posed by the destructive potential inherent in the analytic pursuit of knowledge and truth at all costs, a pursuit that is susceptible to arrogance and perhaps, from the patient's point of view, smacks of omniscience (though Bion does not use this word). In other words, by means of our therapeutic intent and insistent search for truth, we are capable of eliciting a sense annihilation in the patient.

The Analyst's Conundrum

Recognizing this conundrum places the analyst in a bind. Aware that we court disaster through analytic inquiry, should we back off or keep going? Bion expresses a kind of soldierly obligation to carry on with the task, which means working in the trenches without hope of escaping unharmed. Winnicott, writing in this same window of time following World War II, saw a similar danger in the way we apply the analytic search tool to our patients,

DOI: 10.4324/9781032661230-3

though for him the peril springs from interpretations that impinge, thereby exposing the psyche by forcing the patient into premature, explicit communication. Winnicott says:

> We can understand the hatred people have of psychoanalysis which has penetrated a long way into the human personality, and which provides a threat to the human individual in his need to be secretly isolated.
>
> (1965, p. 187)

This prompts Winnicott to ask, "Are we to give up pursuing understanding?", to which his own reply, like Bion's, is to recognize that we must carry on, albeit with an awareness of the inescapable dilemma in which the pursuit of understanding and knowledge can traumatize.

I'm not sure one is supposed to look for a take-away from a Bion paper, but I was left with the impression that the best we can hope for is that our pride in ourselves and our work does not curdle into arrogance, as Bion suggests it can; that we remain humble and willing to identify with the patient, which might lessen the likelihood of falling into a deadly type of arrogant curiosity that can destroy souls in the name of truth-seeking. The question outlined in this brief paper, which also lies at the root of many of Bion's later concerns, is: How might our work lend itself to learning from experience and emotional evolution without subjugating lived experience to the hegemony of a voracious search for instrumental knowledge? (Later in his work, Bion would insist on comparing scientific thought to psychotic thought processes.)

Main Themes and Ideas

"On Arrogance" is in fact about several things, each of which carries quite a payload:

- It presents a distinctive, quasi-psychotic personality structure, which presents itself in the clinical field in the form of scattered references to arrogance, curiosity, and stupidity.
- It describes the workings of an obstructive internal object and its potentially destructive but inevitable implementation in the therapeutic approach of the analyst.
- It introduces the idea of projective identification as a form of primitive communication, and a groundbreaking description of the crucial therapeutic role of the analyst's receptivity and metabolizing function.
- Last but not least, it provides an alternative reading of the Oedipus myth in which it illuminates the psychical dangers of unrestrained knowledge and truth-seeking.

Outline of the Argument

Let me start by following Bion's depiction of these patients in the clinical situation: First, he identifies the presenting picture: a patient who might appear neurotic, but is evidencing negative therapeutic reactions, or at least failing to make progress, but in addition – and this is crucial – displays elements of arrogance, stupidity, and curiosity, though these features, he says, tend to appear in scattered, unrelated fashion. In other words, these features must be noticed by the analyst as belonging together and recognized for what they are – a specific manifestation of an underlying psychical disaster, a ruined psyche. In this way, Bion brings to our attention the existence of a particular kind of psychotic character disorder, or what the neo-Kleinians might call a *pathological organization*, in which the psychotic elements are hidden from view, in this case by means of the dispersal of pathological elements into apparently unrelated forms of arrogance, stupidity, and curiosity. But what seems present here, and absent in the Kleinian model, is Bion's insistence that this type of personality organization is built atop a primitive psychical catastrophe, which might imply the existence of early trauma, or what Winnicott would call *environment failure*. Bion, however, studiously avoids references to early-life explanations, which is consistent with his firmly held position against cause–effect thinking in psychoanalysis. But, while he makes no attempt to identify etiology, it is clear that something terrible has happened to these patients. If the surviving pseudo-normal superstructure might mislead the analyst into treating the patient like a neurotic, the substructure could not be more at variance with that of the neurotic: Bion uses the image of the archeological ruin to picture the underlying psychical reality; the shards and fragments must be pieced together so that the disaster that has occurred can be discerned.

But this is not all. Beyond depicting how this type of post-catastrophe personality presents itself, Bion identifies and provides an original description of the workings of certain primitive psychical mechanisms and processes that predominate in these personalities. These involve, above all, the presence of an *obstructive object* in the inner world, an object that cannot or will not receive and metabolize the projected fragments of the patient's psyche, thus disabling projective identification in its growth-enhancing and therapeutic potential. Indeed, as Larry Brown noted in a recent discussion (personal communication), it is in this brief paper on arrogance that Bion offers the founding statement on the clinical importance of the analyst's receptivity and metabolization of projective identifications – a prelude to the more developed models of *container–contained* and of *alpha function*.

I would note that, along with this initial statement on how the projective identifications are received and tolerated by the analyst, this paper also provides a preliminary outline of the operation of the psychotic part of the personality, which is developed more fully in another paper written at that time,

"Differentiation of the Psychotic from the Non-Psychotic Personalities" (1957), and then in "The Psycho-Analytic Study of Thinking" (1962b) and *Learning from Experience* (1962a), where Bion more clearly contrasts normal and pathological processes of splitting and projective identification. In the psychotic part of the personality, the excessive need to evacuate interferes with the communicative function of projective identification, blocking the crucial ability to take-back-in (useful introjection). Thus, the psychotic process reverses the metabolizing capacities of the mind, replacing alpha function with the beta screen, which operates on the principle of expulsion as a means of psychical survival, hence precluding any learning from experience. Though these concepts were not yet articulated in this 1958 paper on arrogance, the seeds of all of these ideas are there.

To return to the conception of the *obstructive object* as a main feature of these post-catastrophe personalities, the implications for clinical work are illuminating and daunting. Bion describes what it means not only to encounter the existence of the obstructive object in the patient's inner world and behavior, but for the analyst himself to become such an object in the clinical encounter, which he warns is inevitable. What is more, the analyst's entire approach and method are, by their very nature, a provocation – an iatrogenic setup. In the avid pursuit of the psychical truth, analysis itself becomes potentially ego-destructive.

As I have noted, Bion does not describe the clinical encounter with these patients in terms of a repetition of trauma situations or reliving an earlier disaster, as might Ferenczi, or as Winnicott portrays in "Fear of Breakdown" (1974). Instead, Bion takes us into the workings of a mental structure that has been built upon the psychical ruins, a *superstructure*, as it were, which is dominated by this obstructionist object that has the qualities of a primitive superego (which Bion later describes as a kind of *super* Superego, willing to dismantle or destroy the ego). Presumably what sets this organized type of pathological personality organization apart from a more frankly disorganized psychotic picture is precisely this capacity, in certain survivors of trauma, to construct an omniscient superstructure that then serves to mask the underlying fragmentation and splitting in the personality.[1] Somehow, in these cases, a survivalist ego, having risen from the ashes, is capable of constructing a pseudo-normal facsimile of sanity, and this raises what I consider an important question: Is it the tyranny of the obstructive superego object alone that enforces the pathological organization, forcing the ego to follow its dictates under threat of destruction and leaving the ego terrorized and confused? Or has the ego itself become more fully the agent of tyranny, along the lines of identification with the aggressor, or in the form of a sociopathic false-self built on systematic dissociation from human need?

We have seen that this paper is expressly about a certain kind of patient, a person in whom the psychotic elements are active but implicit. This clinical picture approximates something like a pathological organization of the personality taking the form of a psychotic character, or what might be called a post-catastrophic personality. But the implications of Bion's ideas as they are inscribed in this paper go far beyond what we may find in working with any particular type of patient, challenging us to reconsider certain basic assumptions of psychoanalytic practice, or what Civitarese (2020), in his recent, searching article on Bion's "On Arrogance", refers to as the *ideology* of psychoanalysis. It is true that attitudes have changed in many parts of the analytic world: Theoretical certainty, prevalent in Bion's time, has given way to more humble attitudes (owing partly, in some ways, to Bion's own influence). In the US, for example, theoretical pluralism and the intersubjective perspective have replaced the sectarian hegemony of mainstream psychoanalytic belief of forty years ago. Yet, in our daily work with each and every patient, problems of how we deploy knowledge and search for truth remain as challenging and alive as ever. Bion's 1958 paper seems not only prescient but highly relevant to everyday psychoanalytic thought and practice.

The Oedipus Myth Reinterpreted

Nowhere does Bion's paper have a more incendiary impact than in the brief comments on the Oedipus myth. This is how he launches the critique:

> I shall rehearse the Oedipus myth from a point of view which makes the sexual crime a peripheral element of a story in which the central crime is the arrogance of Oedipus in vowing to lay bare the truth at no matter what cost.
>
> (p. 144)

Barely attempting a justification of this insurgent interpretation of the Oedipus story, Bion proceeds by invoking certain characters who feature prominently in the myth, more by way of demonstration than explanation or argument, as if introducing his new reading of Oedipus directly into our dream consciousness:

> The sphinx, who asks a riddle and destroys herself when it is answered, the blind Teiresias, who possesses knowledge and deplores the resolve of the king to search for it, the oracle that provokes the search which the prophet deplores, and again the king who, his search concluded, suffers blindness and exile.
>
> (p. 144)

So, in no more than a couple of short paragraphs, Bion mounts a discreet challenge to a foundational myth of psychoanalysis, reinterpreting the Oedipus myth as an epistemophilic crime of hubris rather than a crime of sex and murder, and does it in such a way as to ignite curiosity and stimulate a flurry of questions about our analytic praxis. (Civitarese, 2020, in his discussion of "On Arrogance", easily spends several pages expanding on Bion's miniaturist treatment of the Oedipus myth, and I would have happily read several more.)

The Fate of Interpretation

Early on in the paper, Bion pinpoints the dilemma posed by working analytically with these patients:

> The analytic procedure itself is precisely a manifestation of the curiosity which is felt to be an intrinsic component of the disaster. As a consequence, the very act of analyzing the patient makes the analyst an accessory in precipitating regression and turning the analysis itself into a piece of acting out.
>
> (p. 144)

Since, as Bion says, this conundrum is unavoidable if we are to carry on doing our work, he suggests that there is nothing for it but to make the best of a bad job, turning the regression and acting out "to good account", as he puts it, by means of:

> Detailed interpretation of events that are taking place in the session. These events are active displays of the mechanisms of splitting, projective identification, and the related subsidiary phenomena of confusional states, depersonalization and hallucination.
>
> (p. 144)

Bion's emphasis here on interpretation would seem consistent with both Freudian and Kleinian approaches, but differs in certain respects: For one thing, Bion recognizes that, in these cases, the transference is to the "analyst as analyst", to the actual person of the analyst as experienced by the patient, rather than the analyst as a mere phantasy construction or representation of a figure from the past. This would lead to interpretations addressed not to uncovering repressed imagoes, but to the mental functioning of the patient in the here and now, and to what is actually going on between analyst and patient in the present. (Civitarese considers this shift towards interpreting in the here-and-now of particular significance in this paper.)

But, despite this new slant in Bion's use of interpretation, he does continue to stress its central role in clinical work. This might reflect Bion's high valuation, evident in his earlier writings, of the patient's attainment of verbal-symbol and thinking capacities, including the capacity for abstraction. This reaches its apotheosis in the concept of alpha function, introduced not long after his writing this paper. Is it fair to say that the later Bion – the Bion of *Transformations* (1967) and *Attention and Interpretation* (1970) – no longer emphasizes the role of interpretation as the main technical approach? Not that he would abandon interpretation, but other things became more prominent in his newer clinical approach – the *container–contained* relation, the *selected fact, transformations in O* – which depend upon the analyst's state of receptivity, reverie, and relinquishment of a mental attitude of knowing. This new clinical perspective began to alter the conception of interpretation – not so much the analyst providing interpretations based on the application of knowledge or insight, but interpretation arising in the clinical field, in the interaction between analyst and patient, as described and richly developed later in the work of Ogden (1999) and of the post-Bionian field theorists (Ferro, 2009). But one can see kernels of many of these later ideas right here, in this early paper "On Arrogance".

Yet, at the same time, there remains something ambiguous or off-kilter about the emphasis in this paper on *interpreting* the mechanism of splitting and projection: Here, in the emphasis on the analyst's interpretive activity, Bion avows a position that seem at odds with the ethos of the new idea he is offering. After all, the brilliant discoveries presented in the paper are all in the direction of recognizing the importance of relinquishing the position of the *one who knows*, as Lacan put it – the importance of stepping aside from the position of interpreter in favor of accepting an identificatory process as the basis for the cure, and shifting the clinical approach to accepting a role in what Bion calls "primitive" communication with the patient. So, when he incongruously reasserts the ultimate primacy of interpretation, it raises the question in my mind: Is this an example of an unprocessed residue of Kleinian thinking? In 1958, Bion was, after all, still very much in the Kleinian fold, and perhaps not yet able to more fully break free. Civitarese (2020) shows how Bion's paper, while at times striking a more characteristically assertive note, is for the most part quite cautious and tentative rather than confrontative in tone and rhetoric. In this way, the radical import of his ideas was perhaps being introduced, to some degree, in stealth fashion.

I am not sure, however, whether this and other statements in the paper do not in fact reflect an enduring element in Bion's thinking, in which the formative effects of the *other* or the *environment*, the traumatizing dimension, tend to take a back seat to the constitutional strength of the destructive death instinct. (This is a point upon which Bion and Winnicott would then truly diverge.) Of course, Bion would soon come to give the greatest importance to the analyst's actual role in processes of containment and transformation, but the question of the analyst's active contribution remains more ambiguous (though it is certainly developed later by Ogden and the field theorists as well as relational analysts). Even in this paper, which distinctly breaks new ground by posing the question of whether the analyst is constantly in danger of seducing the patient into a hubristic search for truth, there remains an ambiguity about whether the analyst is doing this owing to the patient's placing him in that position through projective identification, or whether the analyst is the actual source, the originator of the patient's dilemma. Here, one cannot help but think of Laplanche's (1997) reformulation of the analyst role in terms of seduction, and Winnicott's recognition that, where the patient shows resistance, the source lies in the analyst.

The Obstructive Object

The conception of the obstructive object, another important idea making its debut in the pages of this brief paper, is worthy of further scrutiny. In the course of trying to grasp the nature of this obstructive force, which Bion had said is "sometimes in him, sometimes in me, and sometimes occupied an unknown location", he finally comes to an important insight: The obstructive object, he says, is full of curiosity but at the same time cannot stand to take in projections. He goes on to say:

> What it was that the object could not stand became clearer in some sessions where it appeared that in so far as I, as analyst, was insisting on verbal communication as a method of making the patient's problems explicit, I was felt to be directly attacking the patient's methods of communication. From this it became clear that when I was identified with the obstructive force, what I could not stand was the patient's methods of communication. In this phase my employment of verbal communication was felt by the patient to be a mutilating attack on *his* methods of communication.
>
> (p. 146)[2]

What is *the patient's* method of communication? It is primitive projective identification, Bion says, and continues:

> From this point onwards, it was only a matter of time to demonstrate that the patient's link with me was his ability to employ the mechanism of projective identification. That is to say, his relationship with me and his ability to profit by the association lay in the opportunity to split off parts of his psyche and project them into me.
>
> (p. 146)

"From this point on ..." Here, Bion seems to relocate the source of the obstruction back into the patient, rather than in the mode of communication being used by the analyst. It is the patient's internal obstructive – and ego-destructive – object that the patient then unconsciously seeks to evacuate into the analyst, the reception and metabolization of which Bion now recognizes as crucial to the analytic work. This extraordinary and iconic observation and insight into an unconscious form of primitive unconscious communication have, of course, had a profound impact on how we think about the therapeutic interaction, but, in the context of this paper, there is the question of how the source of obstruction and destruction finds its way back into the patient – which, according to Bion, clears the way forward for the analyst to interpret the patient's use of the processes of splitting and projection.

There is no question but that Bion's discernment of the workings of the obstructive object was of immense conceptual and clinical significance, one that would find further elaboration in his developing ideas about moralism, omnipotent thinking, lying, and what he would later describe in terms of –K. But, in the context of this paper on arrogance, it remains unclear whether the analyst comes to be the proxy for the patient's internal obstructive object, which turns the analyst into someone stupid, destructively curious, and arrogant, or whether it is the analyst, sponsored by the blindly curious tendency of psychoanalysis to arrogantly pursue truth at all costs, who is, after all, the obstructive force, insofar as he pursues the impossible, insists on knowing the truth of the unconscious, and wishes to penetrate the human essence, which surely obliges the patient to become obstructive in turn, both as defense and through identification with the analyst. Bion's (1970) later work does, of course, take up this problem of the analyst's knowingness in a big way, with his formulations on K and O, and the injunction to enter the session without memory and desire. But it remains somewhat uncertain in Bion's work whether the source of obstructive objects lies in defects in the environment or in the endogenous psychical tendency to self-destruction ascribed to the patient's death instinct.

But perhaps this ambiguity is the whole point: Am I wanting to subject this remarkable paper to a *logos* that is, after all, the very problem that the paper illuminates?

On Stupidity

Finally, a note on stupidity in relation to curiosity and arrogance. The three things are quite disparate, making an unlikely and somewhat odd trio. Yet their co-existence in the post-traumatic psyche, as discerned by Bion, rings true. There is nothing much good to say about arrogance – from any angle it's bad news – but curiosity is quite a different matter: It can go either way. Curiosity can be a beautiful thing – one can hardly think of being alive to the world or of learning from experience without it – but it can be destructive too, a means of intruding, insinuating, gaining possession. And, as Civitarese (2020) notes, there is often a thin line between the positive and the toxic forms of curiosity.

But the real dark horse in Bion's account is "stupidity". Being stupid could be viewed as unfortunate – it certainly seems unpromising, but, in the context of this paper, it is clearly treated as part of something destructive and malevolent. I don't think stupidity is in itself necessarily a very bad thing, and can even have its uses: If being a little stupid means not being a know-it-all, it is a forgivable trait. But it does seem a little like the odd-man-out of the triumvirate in this paper. What does Bion mean by stupid? Presumably, it does not refer to any particular lack of intelligence, but it could describe the emotional opacity that grows out of arrogance and wanton curiosity. But why does it get equal billing along with the other two blighted features of the post-catastrophe personality?

One could simply ignore this reference to stupidity as another of Bion's unexplained wild thoughts, except that it invariably turns out that he is on to something, even when he seems to be uttering nothing other than a stray thought. So this is what his reference to stupidity leads me to ask: Could it be that the post-traumatic personality is always marked by a kind of stupor, an organized state of dissociation, a way of living at a remove, in an alter world of sorts – an effect of having being disrupted in the core of one's self-experience, a disruption in what Winnicott called *going-on-being*? In this sense of *being in a stupor*, stupidity would be a manifestation of *hypnoid* rather than *schizoid* mechanisms and would mark the existence of a fixed dissociative regime of alienation from embodied experience (Goldberg, 2020), a pathology of mesmerized self-detachment operating alongside the schizoid processes of splitting and projective identification. While Bion did not, to my knowledge, conceptualize dissociation in its own right (as a phenomenon distinct from splitting), his extraordinary powers of observation might nevertheless have led him to recognize the *effects* of dissociation, and stupidity is perhaps the effect he saw.

Notes

1 While Bion highlights the dispersal of evidence of arrogance, stupidity, and malignant curiosity in certain post-catastrophe patients, it seems to me that we can identify other omnipotent and manic formations of the personality.
2 This extraordinary observation about the sometimes devastating incongruity between analyst's and patient's modes of communication finds startling resonance in Winnicott's remarkable paper "Communicating and Not Communicating Leading to a Study of Certain Opposites" (1963).

References

Bion, W.R. (1957). Differentiation of the psychotic from the non-psychotic personalities. *International Journal of Psychoanalysis* 38: 266–275.
Bion, W.R. (1958). On arrogance. *International Journal of Psychoanalysis* 39: 144–146.
Bion, W.R. (1962a, 2014). Vol. 4. *Learning from Experience*. In The Complete Works of W.R. Bion. London: Routledge.
Bion, W.R. (1962b). The psycho-analytic study of thinking. *International Journal of Psychoanalysis* 43: 306–310.1
Bion, W.R. (1967). Vol. 5. *Transformations*. In The Complete Works of W.R. Bion. London: Routledge.
Bion, W.R. (1970). Vol. 6. *Attention and Interpretation*. In The Complete Works of W. R. Bion. London: Routledge.

Civitarese, G. (2020). The limits of interpretation. A reading of Bion's "On Arrogance". *International Journal of Psychoanalysis.* doi:10.1080/00207578.2020.1827954

Ferro, A. (2009). Transformations in dreaming and characters in the psychoanalytic field. *International Journal of Psychoanalysis* 90: 209–230.

Goldberg, P. (2020). Body–mind dissociation, altered states, and alter worlds. *Journal of the American Psychoanalytic Association* 68: 769–806.

Laplanche, J. (1997). The theory of seduction and the problem of the other. *International Journal of Psychoanalysis*, 78: 653–666.

Ogden, T. (1999). *Reverie and Interpretation: Sensing Something Human.* Northvale, NJ: Aronson/London: Karnac.

Winnicott, D.W. (1965). Communicating and not communicating leading to a study of certain opposites. In *The Maturational Processes and the Facilitating Environment* (pp. 179–192). London: Hogarth Press.

Winnicott, D.W. (1974). Fear of breakdown. *International Review of Psycho-Analysis*, 1: 103–107.

Chapter 3

A Theory of Thinking

Thomas P. Helscher

I'd like to start by describing our challenge in discussing this particular paper (Bion, 1962), which is Bion's most cited work, one of the top ten most cited psychoanalytic papers on PEP, and has been deeply saturated with readings, interpretations, and layers of meaning. It is itself almost an institution or museum piece in psychoanalytic literature. In order to avoid our experience of this 'classic' paper becoming that of the figure Bion describes who is loaded with honors and sinks without a trace, I would ask that we approach this encounter with the paper to the extent possible without memory, desire, or understanding, so that we can experience its startling strangeness with new eyes, with a curiosity that enlivens rather than mutilates. In fact, I will argue that the way Bion approaches this subject demands that we engage in what, as an English major in college, we called 'close reading,' which involved disregarding the author's biographical details and leaving in the background the historical context of the literary work as well the social and political conditions of its production, in order to attempt to engage with what Bion might call its non-sensuous essence, an unsaturated thought that perhaps will become a bit more saturated by the time we are done.

He opens the paper by stating that he is "primarily concerned to present a theoretical system," but he immediately emends this statement. For, unlike a pure theoretical statement, like a philosophical theory, he tells us that this paper will be an "applied theoretical statement," bearing the same relationship to pure theory as applied mathematics has to pure mathematics. The statements in this paper are intended to be to clinical facts what mathematical statements about circles are to "a circle drawn upon paper." As we shall see, this early reference to mathematics is not merely analogical or metaphorical, for what he is already calling our attention to is the relationship between the elements of thought, between preconceptions, conceptions, concepts, and even scientific deductive systems.

For a paper derived supposedly from clinical experiences, our version of 'circles drawn on paper,' however, this is a curiously abstract beginning. He's not calling our attention to a particular patient, as he does, for example, in "On Arrogance," or a particular pathological formulation, such as psychotic

DOI: 10.4324/9781032661230-4

versus non-psychotic parts of the personality, or even particular clinical phenomena, such as "attacks on linking," arrogance, or curiosity. As such, we are already dislocated from our familiar clinical anchoring points of diagnostic categories, case histories, concepts of psychopathology, even metapsychological theory (our field's scientific deductive system). We are therefore forced to begin in a state of not-knowing and uncertainty, relieved only by Bion's assurance that we practicing psychoanalysts will "experience realizations that approximate to the theory." In short, like the situation of the analyst at the beginning of any given analytic session, we are presented initially with an experience of not-knowing, perhaps even frustration, in that we find ourselves confronted with a clinical paper that offers no preexisting clinical signposts or agreed-upon clinical facts. The conceptual space before us seems infinite, minimally saturated with recognizable phenomena. As he will shortly describe, a situation such as this, of not-knowing and an absent object (those missing circles on paper), presents us with a choice of tolerating this difficult feeling long enough to modify it (or have faith that Bion will help us modify it, the crucial intersubjective or social capacity, as it turns out, that I will address at the end of the paper). Or, short of closing the book and throwing it across the room (an impulse I had frequently when I was beginning to 'read' Bion on my own), we could go read what someone else who knows what's going on here has to say about it, for example. There is also a third option, if we can avoid turning away from it altogether, but can't really bear the difficulty long enough to let it evolve into something personally meaningful. This third option he describes as substituting omniscience for thinking. Clearly, for example, we all know what Bion is talking about when he talks about thinking versus evasion or evacuation of the bad feeling, don't we? I would suggest that, whether deliberately or not, Bion's writing almost inevitably poses this epistemological dilemma for us – and we find ourselves fighting the temptation to be seduced by the comfort of someone else's omniscient reading of Bion or any number of what he calls later column-two evasions of emotional contact with reality. I can assure you that those numerous invaluable glosses on this paper are well worth reading carefully, but my point is only that they are not a substitute for the discomforting experience of confronting this strangely and even maddeningly abstract essay.

If we were to consider the larger rhetorical or political effect of this move away from the traditional framework of psychoanalytic writing, we would become aware of two related effects – first, Bion removes himself from debate about psychoanalysis and its theories and directs our attention instead to these hypothetical experiences that he is confident we will recognize from our work with patients. This a not a paper designed to defend, elaborate, extend, or modify preexisting Kleinian or Freudian concepts, although it will make use of some of these concepts where necessary and, in using them, modify them significantly – primarily Freud's two principles of mental functioning and Klein's theory of projective identification. More generally, I would assert then that this paper represents a radical attempt to describe the moment of emotional contact with any reality whatsoever, and how things so often go horribly wrong in that encounter. The second effect then stems from the realization that Bion is boldly reframing the task of psychoanalysis, if not the task of being human, as bearing the pain of existence, and how we develop the capacity to do that in the face of what feels like intolerable pressure – pressure Bion is careful not to situate as either primarily an internal or external problem. I would note that, by not privileging either internal or external factors, he is avoiding the bitter antagonism between the internal phantasy camp of the Kleinians and the environmental camp of the Winnicottians or middle school, as well as presaging his own emphasis on the space between subject and object – the link, the synapse, the caesura. I'd like to highlight the importance, even in this relatively early paper, of the in-between space that we will later come to think of as the field, the intersubjective, the link.

He begins, then, by first describing the emotional experience from which it has been abstracted – the development of thinking out of the pressure generated by the emergence of thoughts. He stresses the sequence here – thoughts precede the development of the "apparatus to cope with them." He points out that problems may arise from either: (1.) a breakdown in the development of thoughts or (2.) a breakdown in the development of the apparatus for dealing with them. The open-endedness of how he describes the source of the problem would seem to suggest the inextricability of innate constitution, the intensity of the experience (which is the place where inner and outer are joined), and the capacity of the container to dampen this intensity. In other words, the problem might arise from either or both container and contained, thoughts and the apparatus for thinking them, and I think it important to hold how both of those are *simultaneously* internal and external phenomena.

He goes on to classify 'thoughts' generally as being preconceptions, conceptions or thoughts, and concepts, seemingly using the term 'thought' here to characterize mental phenomena in general, a commonsense use of the term. He then describes this process of the development of 'thoughts,' from the empty thought of the preconception – there is a breast or an analyst or a need-satisfying object out there somewhere, waiting to be found – to the fate of that preconception at the moment of contact with reality, and the two different outcomes possible. (Of course, if we're beginning to get the sense of this thinking in terms of non-linear complexity that he seems to be stimulating in us, we might wonder why only two, why not an infinite spectrum of possibilities between these two poles of satisfaction and frustration?) First, a positive experience of fulfillment or satisfaction, in which the preconception is met, or, second, a negative experience if the preconception is not met: "The model I propose is that of an infant whose expectation of a breast is mated with a realization of no breast available for satisfaction. This mating is experienced as a no-breast, or 'absent' breast inside."

I would like us to pause for a second and contemplate the dizzying leap Bion has just described in this model of the infant's experience of frustration. When the expectation – a preconception in Bion's terminology – that a desire or need will be fulfilled is not satisfied, the feeling of non-satisfaction can become a 'thing,' a 'no breast' or 'absent breast inside.' Of course, from a post-Kleinian or Bionian perspective, we 'know' what this means – the formation in the mind of the first bad object out of the libidinally bad experience of pain, a phenomenon both Klein and Fairbairn wrote extensively about. However, from within the model he's proposing, there is as yet no mind available in which to register this object – the apparatus for thinking thoughts is developed post hoc in response to this hypothetical moment of painful experience. So, if the Christian version of this originary moment is "in the beginning was the word, and the word was with God and the word was God," for Bion, it might be, in the beginning was the shock of pain, and the pain became a thing that might (or might not) become a thought.

Now, at this point in the paper, in a critical moment of definitory hypothesis, Bion restricts the general meaning of thoughts as all the mental phenomena he described above to this specific experience of non-satisfaction that creates the 'no thing.' Everything in the paper that follows stems from this restriction of 'thoughts' to the non-sensuous experience of frustration or 'no thing.' So, curiously, the evolution of 'thought' does not track through the satisfying experience of fulfillment which produces a conception, and then through repeated iterations of concepts, and so on, but must pass through this uncertain and painful path of frustration and dissatisfaction. As he goes on to describe, the outcome of this experience of the 'first thought' is uncertain and depends upon what he describes somewhat frustratingly as "the infant's capacity for frustration: in particular it depends on whether the decision is to evade frustration or to modify it." I would just point out a particular fudge at this point in his reasoning – since he seems to describe the issue as one of 'capacity' at this originary moment of mindlessness, we have to wonder, 'capacity of what?' The infant's neurological system, its proto-mental matrix, its sturdiness of constitution, whatever that might mean? And yet he says it depends in particular on a 'decision.' Who or what, if there is no mental apparatus yet, is doing the deciding? Is it possible the infant's capacity might include an Other who is intimately involved in both 'the capacity' and the 'decision'? I believe this is so and that this will become clearer as his thought develops over the course of the paper. (Of course, at this point, it's hard not to think of Winnicott's thought that there is no infant without a mother.)

From this point on, his description of the process becomes somewhat more straightforward: "If the capacity for frustration is sufficient the 'no breast' inside becomes a thought and an apparatus for 'thinking' it develops." One wonders how the "no breast" object becomes a thought if the apparatus for thinking it is an effect of it becoming a thought rather than the cause of it becoming a thought. We will have to sit with that question or paradox for a moment, because, again, I think it will become (only) somewhat clearer by the end of the paper.

At this point, Bion differentiates between the mature personality (or mature aspect of the personality) who is already capable of recognizing a bad object as a thought and the immature personality (or immature aspect of the personality) who is confronted with "the need to decide between evasion of frustration or of its modification." I would suggest that we should 'think' of this 'moment' as more simultaneous and less developmental and linear – at any moment there is a part of the personality we might call mature or neurotic capable of recognizing a thought and an immature or undeveloped (emergent) aspect of the personality that is confronted with the need to evade or modify frustration. We could link this simultaneity of mental experience to Bion's work with groups – the basic assumption group and the workgroup exist and evolve simultaneously, or at least potentially exist simultaneously. This non-linear understanding of psychic experience seems both an extension of Freud's work on the dynamic relationship between the repressed and timeless unconscious and the linear and more rational conscious mind, the primary and secondary process paper Bion references here, as well of Klein's work with positions rather than linear developmental stages, and also a preconception or early understanding of quantum physics and its concepts of superposition and Heisenberg's uncertainty principle.

What I find clinically important at this point is that Bion is focusing our attention on the moment of emergence and maximal uncertainty – the point where the immature aspects of the personality confront an experience that threatens to overwhelm and profoundly disorganize it. It is worth noting that the problem is defined in terms of capacity to bear frustration rather than something such as innate envy, destructiveness, or aggression – that is, Klein's constitutional death drive. Instead of 'becoming' a thought – the product of a juxtaposition of a preconception and negative realization – it becomes a bad object, indistinguishable from a thing-in-itself, fit only for evacuation. Or, as my first control case described the situation repeatedly and with deep resignation, "it is what it is" – that is, inert, a thing, resistant to being transformed into a thought and submitted to alpha function (or is it alpha function that transforms it into a thought?). The result is a "hypertrophic development of the apparatus for projective identification" in which evacuation of the bad breast "is synonymous with obtaining sustenance from a good breast." Here, Bion seems to be referencing Freud's description of the pleasure/unpleasure principle, in which the reduction of unpleasurable stimulation is equivalent to pleasure.

Curiously, at this point, he turns the discussion to "mathematical elements," which derive from "realizations of two-ness as in breast and infant, two eyes, two feet and so on." At first blush, this seems a startling insertion of abstraction into the phenomenological description of this origin of thought out of barely tolerated frustration versus projective identification, and yet what we are in fact witnessing is the emergence into the field of the Other – and the dyad that exists as preconception in projective identification. A projection requires a space into which the projection is sent that contains it, a point Bion will elaborate in great detail in *Transformations*. (As my colleague Afsaneh Alisobhani has kindly pointed out to me, Bion takes the concept of 'realization' from a book he was studying at this time entitled *Algebraic Projective Geometry*, which traces the emergence of three-dimensional models of algebraic geometry out of the two-dimensional geometry of Euclid – the geometry of circles drawn on paper. This text provides Bion with the concepts of rigid motion and projective transformations he will explore in *Transformations*.) The experience or 'realization' of two-ness then opens the way to 'modification' of frustration. The ability of the infant or the immature aspects of the personality to experience two-ness that is characteristic of projective identification allows then for "the development of conceptions" in the absence of satisfying experience. Perhaps more accurately, the experience of two-ness in projective identification – the realization of the preconception of two-ness – provides the satisfying experience of mental or emotional containment, if not the bodily satisfaction of real milk. This distinction is critical – Bion is suggesting that the non-sensuous 'satisfaction' of mental containment is equivalent to physiological satisfaction but in a different register as it were. It is emotional containment and not the experience of physiological satisfaction that represents the origins of thinking.

If the intolerance of frustration is too great, however, the capacity to experience this 'realization of two-ness' is compromised by excessive projective identification. As Bion observes, "the dominance of projective identification confuses the distinction between the self and the external object." This *excessive* projective identification destroys the preconception necessary for the experience of external reality – Kant's a priori categories of space and time. As he poignantly goes on to describe,

> the relationship with time was graphically brought home to me by a patient who said over and over again that he was wasting time – and continued to waste it. The consequences are illustrated in the description in *Alice in Wonderland* of the Mad Hatter's tea-party – it is always four o'clock.

In this singular clinical vignette, the only reference in this paper to an actual patient and a real clinical experience, Bion illustrates how excessive projection identification destroys the preconceptions of time and space that make possible our capacity to turn the world of things-in-themselves, the noumenal, into our subjective experiences or phenomena. I want to emphasize that Bion is here equating excessive projective identification with the destruction of the necessary preconception of two-ness that makes projective identification itself possible.

As he will make explicit later in the paper, the sequence of the development of the capacity to think rests on this originary preconception of two-ness – what he describes elsewhere as the innate preconception of a need-fulfilling object. And here is where he radically revises Klein's theory of projective identification, which is ultimately always a phantasy, the projection into an internal object, admittedly one which has real consequences on the inter-subjective field. As in the case he describes in "On Arrogance," projective identification – the emotional communication of unmentalized emotional experience – is the necessary precursor to the development of the capacity to think thoughts. This is not a psychopathological condition but is, in fact, necessary to the development of our capacity to bear the emergence of a thought out of a painful experience of absence or frustration. When, for example, as in the case he describes in "On Arrogance," the analyst/mother cannot tolerate the projective identification, development of thinking ceases, and, as in the Mad Hatter's tea party, time and space are suspended, and it is always 4 o'clock.

At this point, Bion distinguishes between the damaging effects of excess of belief in omnipotence and the capacity to tolerate modification through pro-jective identification. As an example of this destructive potential of excessive belief in omnipotence, he offers the phantasy of treating the realization of two-ness as if it were "indistinguishable from things-in-themselves and ... evacuated at high speed as missiles to annihilate space." Or, to put it more simply, aspects of projective identification, specifically its evacuative potential, are weaponized and used to destroy the necessary substrate of reality in Kantian terms – the grid of time and space. I'll pose a question at this point that perhaps we can return to later: is this moment of annihilation of time and space also a constant aspect of our experience, at least momentarily? Something that breaks up the continuous flow of our unconscious narrative of self, and not merely a pathological mechanism characteristic of only the most disturbed patients? I think this question points to the tension in this paper between the psychopathological Kleinian thinker and the emerging mystic of *Transformations* and *Attention and Interpretation*.

In contrast to this excessive projective identification, he offers normal pro-jective identification as the necessary precursor to communication:

> as a realistic activity it [projective identification] shows itself as a beha-
> viour reasonably calculated to arouse in the mother feelings of which the
> infant wishes to be rid; if the infant feels that it is dying it can arouse
> fears in the mother that it is dying.

Thus, the realization of two-ness, if not destroyed by omnipotent attacks on the foundations of our experience – time and space – allows for an inter-subjective exchange, not merely in the internal world of the infant, but in the space between infant and mother – a space created by the mating of the infant's preconception of two-ness with the mother's alpha function. In good non-linear fashion, Bion attributes breakdowns in this dyadic process of 'normal' projective identification not solely to the incapacity of the infant to 'tolerate frustration,' but also to the mother's capacity to "accept these [projections] and respond therapeutically." For, "if the mother cannot tolerate these projections, the infant is reduced to continued projective identification carried out with increasing force and frequency." At the risk of belaboring the point, in this complex and dynamic exchange, we can't simply say it is the incapacity of the infant or his predilection for omnipotence that creates the problem; as with the obstructive object Bion describes in "On Arrogance," this object is co-created by subject and object and is both the cause and effect of the collapse of 'the realization of two-ness.' The demand Bion makes on us at this moment to me resembles what Winnicott describes as the paradox that must be tolerated and not resolved. We can't say which came first, the omnipotent egg or the projective identification-rejecting chicken. But what we can describe are the meaning-destroying effects of this situation – "the increased force seems to denude the projection of its penumbra of meaning." I think what he means here is that intensity undampened by maternal reverie strips the experience of potential for thoughts to evolve into something tolerable, and the increasing intolerability leads to more and more evacuative processes. Instead of the proliferation of alpha elements that create a kind of ozone layer he describes in *Learning from Experience* as the contact barrier, we get the deterioration of the emotional atmosphere and the increasingly destructive intensity of direct solar radiation.

Since we are in a pre- or proto-mental state of mind, there is no alpha function, except that supplied by the mother, and therefore no contact barrier separating conscious into unconscious and "convert[ing] sense data into alpha elements, and thus provid[ing] the psyche with the material for dream thoughts and hence the capacity to wake up or go to sleep, to be conscious or unconscious." At this stage, the infant (or infantile or undeveloped aspect of personality) is able to:

> produce 'sense data' of the self but ... there is no alpha function to convert them into alpha elements and therefore permit of a capacity for being conscious or unconscious of the self. The infant personality by itself is unable to make use of the sense-data, but has to evacuate these elements into the mother, relying on her to do whatever has to be done to convert them into a form suitable for employment by the infant as alpha-elements.

I just want to underscore the paradigm shift Bion is introducing here – this is not pathological development but absolutely essential to normal development of the capacity to think and feel one's own experience and, therefore, to develop a sense of self. This is not about destructiveness but about survival in a state of overwhelm. There is no mention in this paper of envy or hatred. There is a description of destructive attacks designed to eliminate something that is felt to be unbearable. And he is describing not simply the state of the infant, but the state of all of us in every moment, to a greater or lesser extent – seeking alpha function and containment of potentially unbearable distress.

At this point, anyone familiar with Bion knows what comes next. In his most famous passage, in an uncharacteristically poetic and evocative metaphor, Bion describes the normal (as opposed to excessive) experience of projective identification:

> Normal development follows if the relationship between infant and breast permits the infant to project a feeling that it is dying into the mother and reintroject it after its sojourn in the breast has made it tolerable to the infant psyche. If the projection is not accepted by the mother, the infant feels that its feeling that it is dying is stripped of such meaning as it has [the penumbra of potential associations, preconceptions, proto-mental phenomena, including the vital preconception of two-ness and its realization]. It therefore reintrojects not a fear of dying made tolerable, but a nameless dread.

I think it important to note that this 'nameless dread' is not a bounded and represented thought, but an infinite sense of overwhelm. I think we are in the state he later describes as O, the void and formless infinite, from which thoughts must be won.

At this point in the paper, Bion takes up the outcome of this intersubjective failure and, I believe, turns toward what will preoccupy him for the rest of his career – the elaboration of the primitive defenses against the overwhelm of the "void and formless infinite." The problem is not thinking thoughts on which we have some satisfying purchase (our prior understanding of Bion's thinking, for example); it is tolerating the 'void and formless infinite' from which thoughts emerge. Certainly, this struggle will preoccupy him in *Transformations* and *Attention and Interpretation*. I think he is reaching for a model of mind that begins with a traumatic confrontation with reality in the form of thoughts that one cannot yet think.

He states: "the apparatus available to the psyche may be regarded as fourfold," explicitly not limiting that description to the infant psyche or the pathological psyche. I would suggest that what he is describing here are the always-present, undeveloped or immature aspects of the personality that have not yet been contained by alpha function, whether one's own or the analyst's/mother's. And I would argue that not only is he describing this experience, he is enacting it in the text at this moment. The process of normal development, via projective identification and its breakdown and the consequences of that failure, seems clearly and even beautifully described. Clear enough. We have a sound conception of, and now – some sixty years later – a sturdy concept for, what he's describing up to this point. We seem to have some degree of closure and clarity, and, if we wanted a thumbnail sketch of Bion for Beginners, it would stop here. In fact, the only two comments he makes about this paper in the commentary bear directly, if characteristically enigmatically, on this resistance to closure and the neatness of a satisfying theoretical statement.

He now returns to where he began, not to summarize but to expand and tease out the sensuous and bodily experience of distress from the purely mental non-sensuous: the moment of overwhelm under the pressure and the demand brought to bear by thoughts in their non-sensuousness. Thoughts are not simply the evolved form of 'sense data.' He takes great pains to define thoughts as different from the elaboration of bodily sensations, although these non-sensuous thoughts and sense data from the body are subjected to the same process of what he calls "publication, communication, and common sense" (which he later describes less confusingly as "correlation"). He concludes the paper by drawing parallels between the role of sensory data – the experience of a body in space and time – and the non-sensuous experience of emotions, while still preserving the distinction between purely sensory aspects and non-sensuous or psychic elements. These 'thoughts,' just like sense data, have to be "modified and worked on by alpha-function to make them available for dream-thoughts."

He turns then to the problem of 'publication,' which he defines as making "private awareness (that is awareness that is private to the individual) public." At this point he asserts, seemingly out of nowhere, the essentially social nature of humans: "The emotional problems are associated with the fact that the human individual is a political animal and cannot find fulfillment outside a group and cannot satisfy any emotional drive without expression of its social component." He poses the problem: how do we balance our narcissistic experience of our singularity as an entity occupying a body in a particular moment in time and space with our need to satisfy "any emotional drive" through an expression of its social component? We find ourselves back with the preconception and realization of two-ness, only this time with an emphasis on its non-sensuous dimension:

> In its origins communication is effected by realistic projective identification ... It may develop, if the relationship with the breast is good, into a capacity for toleration by *the self of its own psychical qualities*, and so pave the way for alpha-function and normal thought. But it does also develop as a part of the social capacity of the individual. *This development, of great importance in group dynamics, has received virtually no attention; its absence would make even scientific communication impossible* [italics added].

I think this point of our group constitution as thinkers might explain why Bion demands to be read and discussed in groups, and why simply reading him on one's own can be unbearably frustrating and unrewarding. It's like trying to use Euclidean geometry to solve problems that require three or more dimensions.

We've moved very quickly from the primitive and rudimentary communication of projective identification between the infant and its mother to the social and scientific situation we find ourselves in today at this workshop. A dizzying leap from the two- to the three-dimensional – from Euclidean to projective geometry. I believe that this movement is made possible by Bion insisting on the parallel realms of the sensuous and the non-sensuous that he is here reserving for thought – which I would argue is precisely the thought he is trying to think in this paper. In the Commentary to *Second Thoughts* (1967), Bion describes this thought in some detail, using the language he developed in *Transformations*:

> For a proper understanding of the situation when attacks on linking are being delivered, it is useful to postulate thoughts that have no thinker. I cannot here discuss the problems, but need to formulate them for further investigation, thus: Thoughts exist without a thinker. The idea of infinitude is prior to any idea of the finite. The finite is "won from the dark and formless infinite". Restating this more concretely, the human personality is aware of infinity [is the infant's feeling that it is dying a manifestation of this "awareness of infinity"?]. It becomes aware of limitation, presumably through physical and mental experience of itself and the sense of frustration [is this the effect of the mother's reverie turning infinite experience into the frustration of hunger or the bodily discomfort of cold, clammy wetness?]. A number that is infinite, a sense of infinity, is replaced, say by a sense of threeness. The sense that an infinite number of objects exists is replaced by a sense that only three objects exist; infinite space becomes finite space. The thoughts which have no thinker acquire, or are acquired by a thinker.

And yet, this is not an end point, a permanent developmental milestone, but simply a moment in a dynamic flux between thoughts we can have come to think and thoughts without a thinker that we must wrest from the void and formless infinite.

I think we are brought back once again to the very curious definition of thoughts in this paper. He titles the paper "A Theory of Thinking" (1962) but describes thinking as a process that is necessitated by the impingement of thoughts – in all of their non-sensuous formlessness. And this impingement is constant and inextricable from being alive and emotionally connected to others. Thoughts are reserved for those experiences of gap or lack or, to be more precise, what can arise out of the gap or lack – what can be won from the void and formless infinite, if we can tolerate that seemingly infinite moment of wordless, terrifying, unbearable overwhelm. There is never a point at which we are not subject to that moment (although we may comfort ourselves with the illusion of knowing and being in a closed system).

I think we can see Bion wrestling in this paper to free himself from the restrictive confines of much of psychoanalytic thinking at this time, with its biological, medical, and metapsychological certainties and rigidities. In his one explicit critique of this paper in the Commentary (1967), his one 'second thought' about it, he describes the illusory sense of security of the scientist working within such a closed scientific deductive system:

> I would warn against the phrase, "empirically verifiable data" which I employ in 100. I do not mean that experience 'verifies' or 'validates' anything. This belief as I have come across it in the literature of the philosophy of science relates to an experience which enables the scientist to achieve a feeling of security to offset and neutralize the sense of the insecurity following on discovery that discovery has exposed further vistas of unsolved problems – 'thoughts' in search of a thinker.

What Bion has placed at the center of this paper are precisely thoughts that trouble us into thinking, which are not to be conflated with physical sense data. What I hope I have done today is expose "further vistas of unsolved problems" posed by this dense and difficult work.

As a final aside stimulated by the writing of this paper, I would to like to mention (and I would urge you to read) Jacqueline Rose's piece in *The Guardian* recently, entitled "Life after Death: How the Pandemic Has Transformed Our Psychic Landscape" (2021). In it, she describes how the pandemic has forced us collectively, as a species, to face the 'thought' of death and therefore to learn to think together the possibility of collective annihilation:

> We are being robbed of the illusion that we can predict what will happen in the space of a second, a minute, an hour or a day. From one moment to the next, the pandemic seems to turn and point its finger at anyone, even those who believed they were safely immune. ... Nobody knows, with any degree of certainty what will happen next. Anyone claiming to do so is a fraud. ... What on Earth then, we might ask, does the future consist of once the awareness of death passes a certain threshold and breaks into our waking dreams? If the uncertainty strikes at the core of inner life, it also has a political dimension. Every claim for justice relies on a belief in a possible future, even when – or rather especially when – we feel the planet may be facing its demise ... Seen in this light, the relentless drive to push ourselves on and on, as if our lives depended on it – killing us more likely – reveals itself as a doomed effort to bypass inner pain. ... There is a limit to how much we can psychically tolerate. This remains the fundamental insight of psychoanalysis, never more needed than today.

And yet, it seems Bion ends this paper on thinking with the suggestion that we have to continually push up against the limit of what we can psychically tolerate, so that we can learn to think together, collectively, the seemingly unthinkable.

References

Bion, W.R. (1962). A theory of thinking. Published as The psychoanalytic study of thinking. *International Journal of Psycho-analysis,* 43: 306–310.

Bion, W.R. (1967). Commentary. In Vol. 6, *Second Thoughts* (p. 62). The Complete Works of W.R. Bion. London: Routledge.

Rose, Jacqueline (2021). Life after Death: How the Pandemic Has Transformed Our Psychic Landscape. *The Guardian.*

Chapter 4

Differentiation of the Psychotic from the Non-Psychotic Personality

A Link between Early and Late Bion

Afsaneh Kiany Alisobhani

Seminal papers, such as "Differentiation of the Psychotic from the Non-Psychotic Personalities" (Bion, 1957), "like certain works of art, rouse powerful feelings and stimulate growth *willy-nilly*" (Bion, 1967, p. 156, italics added). In Bion's (1967) commentary on *Second Thoughts*, he advises readers that the best of psychoanalytic papers – Freud's and Klein's, to which I would certainly add those of Bion – must be read and then "*forgotten*". "Only in this way is it possible to produce the conditions in which when it is next read, it can stimulate the evolution of further development" (p. 156). His concern was that the power of successful psychoanalytic papers may stimulate a *defensive* reading (*of what the paper is* about) as a *substitute for experiencing* the paper itself, a transformation in K as opposed to a transformation in O. I have read this paper numerous times, discussed it with colleagues and heard several rich commentaries by fellow analysts over the years. The task of "*forgetting*" is not so easy. It is difficult not to read it *defensively*.

However, in my current rereading of "Differentiation of the Psychotic from the Non-Psychotic Personalities" (Bion, 1957), I recognized the seeds of many of Bion's later ideas – the container–contained model, the contact barrier, caesura, and K, L, and H links – that he cultivated and developed in his later work (Bion, 1962, 1963, 1965, 1966, 1970). And I was reminded of the last paragraph of Bion's last paper written in 1979, "Making the Best of a Bad Job" (Bion, 1987a), in which he made a powerful plea to not use his ideas as a barrier to further development and evolution of psychoanalysis. This plea reflected Bion's own position as a disciple of both Freud and Klein, their "heir in the development of the psychoanalytic understanding of psychosis" (see Aguayo, 2016).

In the "Differentiation of the Psychotic from the Non-Psychotic Personalities" (1957), Bion, a Freudian at heart, reread the "Formulations Regarding the Two Principles in Mental Functioning" and Melanie Klein's 1946 paper "Notes on Some Schizoid Mechanisms", weaving through them a creative model for understanding and working with psychosis.

Bion drew a lot from Freud's 1911 paper, but also offered his own modification to the two principles of mental functioning. For Freud, the mother

DOI: 10.4324/9781032661230-5

serves as the aim of the infant's drive discharges. In the absence of such an object to receive them, the infant resorts to hallucinatory wish fulfillment. In the footnote of this paper, he describes the process:

> It probably hallucinates the fulfillment of stimulus and in the absence of satisfaction, by the motor discharge of screaming and beating about with its arms and legs, and it then experiences the satisfaction it has halluci-nated. Later, as an older child, it learns to employ these manifestations of discharge *intentionally* as methods of expressing its feelings.
>
> (Freud, 1911, p. 220)

Action, at the behest of the pleasure principle, is the first thought. Anyone who has watched a baby suckling at the breast will have observed that it is suckling even when the breast is no longer there. The baby continues the *action*, even in the absence of the breast. This *action* is simultaneous with the hallucination of the experience; it is the beginning of thought and the budding of the awareness of its senses; it includes attention, the memory traces left behind, and judgment – a proto-mental thought.

As the pressure of reality builds up, finding that the mother/breast is not there for the discharge of the unpleasure of hunger, the infant must rely on its painful sensory experiences and integrate the consciousness that is attached to them. Freud makes a point that, as the infant grows an *awareness* of the distressing confrontation with the reality principle, it has two ways of dealing with it by way of its drive discharges. If the *frustra-tion* overwhelms it, it can resort to *action* and discharge the accumulation of the stimuli inside somatically. Thinking happens when the infant takes the other route – that is, when, in the absence of satisfaction, the infant postpones the process of discharge and restrain itself from *action*.

Bion was impressed by the idea that thinking always implies absence, a *minus*. He was also intrigued by the notion of *action* and *frustration*. Bion, who primarily thought of himself as a clinician, posed a simple, yet profound question. If a patient was smiling, crying, frowning, looking at the analyst, averting his eyes, or even talking – was the patient communicating? Or was he trying to unburden himself from the unpleasure, and the *consciousness* of the unpleasure? Was he using his ego functions, attention, memory, judgment, in the service of the pleasure principle or reality principle? Or both? Or some-where along that continuum? In his paper "Evidence" (Bion, 1987b), Bion poses the clinical implication of the issue:

> Supposing we are in fact always dealing with some kind of psychoso-matic condition. Is it any good talking to a highly articulate person in a highly articulate term? Is it possible that, if feelings of intense fear, self-hatred, can seep up into a state of mind in which they can be translated

into *action,* the reverse is true? Is it possible to talk to the soma in such a way that the psychosis is able to understand, or vice versa?

(p. 246)

Bion disagreed with Freud on two points. He believed that there is always an *awareness* of the reality principle, however rudimentary, from the very beginning of life. Drawing on Kant's notion of a priori, he used the term preconception as its equivalent and suggested that the baby is born with a preconception – not only of his mother's breast, but also of emotional contact with her mind. If the infant feels its mother's emotional presence, there is an experience of *approximate* positive *realization.* If the mother *frustrates* – for example, if she is dutiful but incapable of reverie, or if she is neglectful or cruel, there is *negative realization.* Wish fulfillment, for Bion, is the *approximation* of *positive realization* of an emotional link with the breast/mother – in Winnicottian language, you might call that a *good enough positive realization.*

If there have been enough cycles of that *good enough positive realization,* depending on the baby's constitution in the context of the mother's capacities, some degree of frustration for the pain of the absent breast is tolerated. The *minus,* the negative realization, the no-breast becomes a thought. The process of positive/negative realization (because mostly *approximately positive*) allows the baby to develop a greater degree of tolerance of *frustration.*

Bion broadened the complexity of the notion of *frustration. Frustration* is the experiential counterpart of the survival instincts in animals. In thermodynamics, a closed system is defined as a system/organism where, even if there is a flow of energy between the organism and the environment, the organism remains unchanged. By contrast, a bacterium's or a virus's DNA, for example, is an open system; it adapts to the demands of the environment, and the adaptation becomes a part of its DNA, causing it to mutate. The human infant's mind is another example of an open system. Humberto Maturana (1999), a Chilean biologist and philosopher, describes adaptation as a constant relation in which organisms and structures change and transform one another *congruently.* When transformation is no longer congruent in the organism and the system, the organism dies. The human DNA is a closed system, but the mind, a biological organism, is an open system. For the human infant, adaptation is the result of learning from experience. The transformational process that is grounded in memory traces of the external and the *link* to the internal reality thus grows capacity for abstract, complex thinking.

Frustration and *realization* are complex processes with a *spectrum* of emergent possibilities. The infant's positive *realization* of the expectation of the breast can only be an approximation – there are many factors that contribute to the gap – pain, envy, greed, hate, the constitutional threshold of the individual, to name a few; but there are infinite factors that are unknown. Tolerating the incompleteness and the imperfection – of the *realization* of the anticipation – yields a spectrum of responses in the face of the *frustration* that ensues.

Bion had another important point of disagreement with Freud. Bion did not accept Freud's dichotomous formulation of the pleasure and reality principles. He hypothesized that the pleasure and reality principles *also* coexist in a *spectrum*. At the end of the "Differentiation" paper, he felt that he was able to clinically substantiate his position.

In this paper, one of Bion's major contributions is his detailed clinical elucidation of the splitting process in the paranoid-schizoid position and the depressive position in the psychotic part of the personality. In the paranoid-schizoid position, the infant makes big splits; it splits the breast into *good* or *bad*, and the nascent ego into *innocent* or *demonic*. Klein views this split as a "division between love and hate" (Klein, 1946). The splitting process in the early stages of development mitigates the overwhelming anxieties faced by the infant. The projective and introjective mechanisms of the internal and external objects lay the foundation for ego and superego development.

The non-psychotic part of the personality is capable of tolerating not only the *frustration* of the negative *realizations*, but also the incomplete, imprecise positive *realization* that fosters the capacity for tolerating time, thus allowing the ability to tolerate space. Time and space make mourning and loss possible, leading to depressive position and the capacity for verbal thought and reflection. Verbalization makes room for assumption of responsibility and guilt.

In the paranoid-schizoid position, when the psychotic mechanism is dominant, the infant minutely splits the parts of its personality that gets it in touch with reality. For the psychotic, owing to its overwhelming destructive impulse and intolerance of frustration, there is a "hatred of reality, internal and external", and a hatred of *awareness* of reality, which makes the normal splitting process impossible. Bion returns to Freud's pleasure/reality principles and says that the psychotic patient not only attacks his consciousness and his sense impressions, but also the elements which could make him conscious *of* his sense impressions. Simultaneously, he also splits his objects into minute particles. The fragments of his ego and the objects are expelled and lodged in the external reality. An awareness of the senses that ordinarily helped him "materially" to establish contact with reality is split off from the senses themselves. For example, seeing and observing are split from the sense of sight, hearing is split from the auditory, and sense of touch is split from skin, resulting in an impairment in attention, memory, judgment, and thought – what Freud considered to be the factors of the ego function.

Moreover, "The foundation of intuitive understanding of himself and others are jeopardized at the outset" (Bion, 1957, p. 47). Perplexed by the caesura of birth, Bion presents an imaginative "fiction" of a fetus's moment of birth in his paper "Evidence" (1987b). He imagines the infant moving from the liquid environment of the womb to the gaseous, fluid world of air. But Bion's is not the sentimental womb of perfect bliss – it is also a place of turbulence and threat. In the presence of all the turmoil – environmental or constitutional – the fetus might choose to get rid of it all. Bion writes:

Suppose this foetus is also aware of the pressures of what will one day turn into a character or a personality, aware of things like fear, hate, crude emotions of that sort. Then the foetus might omnipotently turn its hostility towards these disturbing feelings, proto-ideas, proto-feelings, fragment them, and try to evacuate them. ... I can imagine the foetus being so precocious, so premature that it tries to get rid of its personalities to start off with, and then after birth – still being highly intelligent.

(p. 245)

Frustration is at the foundation of the psychotic part of the personality. Excessive *frustration* gives rise to unbearable pain, psychic pain. It is the psychic pain that hates the awareness of external or internal reality and attacks the apparatus of thinking. The attacks that mutilate the *link* between the external and internal reality and the senses are terrifying – they give rise to a fear of annihilation, which is worse than death itself. It is worse than death, because, when a psychotic mechanism is dominant, the infant is in an infinite void, existence is erased. The defense of the psychotic personality is to collapse time and space. The *links* to the internal and external reality are now fragile. Relationships are precipitate and immature – they vanish as quickly as they appear.

All those fragments – remnants of sense and ego functions and the *links* that attach them to consciousness – are expelled and lodged into external objects. They either penetrate or encyst the objects, and a rudimentary container–contained is formed.

In the depressive position, filled with rage and annihilation anxiety, the psychotic part of the mind tries to restore the mutilated ego, to reestablish *a link*, precociously and hastily, with reality. However, since, through the mechanism of projective identification, the patient has ejected his awareness of his senses, instead of synthesis and integration of the split-off parts, the psychotic agglomerates and arbitrarily compresses the fragments. For example, his sense of sight is now lodged in a gramophone that is now able to spy on him. The patient finds himself trapped in a world populated by what Bion called bizarre objects. Bizarre objects, the split-off aspects of the ego among them, are stripped of their meaning and vitality. They are transformed into things that are endowed with the patient's sadistically harsh, superego. Bion suggests that, where the non-psychotic part of the personality moves in a "dream world", the psychotic part moves in a world of bizarre objects, analogous to the "furniture of dreams" for the non-psychotic part.

Referring to the work of Hannah Segal, Bion suggests that, in the depressive position, forced by the needs of the ego for reparation, the psychotic part of the mind faces an overwhelming fear that it won't survive the depressive anxieties and the profound sadness of the loss of vitality. The psychotic resorts back to the fragmentation of the paranoid-schizoid position. In the paranoid-schizoid position, fragmentation and bizarre objects proliferate and widen the gap between the psychotic and the non-psychotic parts of the mind.

For thinking to develop out of this situation, the ego's repair involves the use of the preverbal elements of the ego. The attacks from the psychotic part of the mind sever the link between sense impressions and the awareness of them. All the psychotic part has as its disposal are the bizarre objects that contain the mangled and stripped-off remnant pieces of his personality and objects that are chaotically compressed and agglomerated for introjection. He then introjects them in the same way they were ejected – what Bion calls projective identification in reverse.

My colleague, Robin Goldberg, who works with profoundly traumatized and autistic children, shared a clinical vignette with me that offers a window into what I have tried to describe. She saw an abused little boy in the therapy room of a preschool. In this session, the little boy saw the lights coming through the partition and thought that they were eyes. Frightened, he bolted out of the room. Dr. Goldberg ran after him and caught him, held him – but he couldn't see her, hear her. Everything was fragmented, including the therapist. Robin held him as he kicked and screamed, and then he relaxed – and the wildness went out of his eyes, and he saw her. "It's me, Dr. Robin, It's just me." They went back into the playroom hand in hand. Later, Dr. Goldberg reports, at around ten years of age, he had episodes of pyromania, which is a vivid illustration of the projective identification in reverse.

In "Neurosis and Psychosis" (1924), Freud does not elaborate on how, in psychosis, the ego reconciles the conflict with external reality. He simply offers a possible scenario and writes "it will be possible for the ego to avoid a rupture in any direction by deforming itself, by submitting to encroachments on its own unity and even perhaps by affecting *a cleavage or division of itself*" (pp. 152–153, italics added). In the "Psychotic" paper, while Bion devotes most of the paper to describing the workings of the psychotic part of the mind, he also emphasizes that there is always a non-psychotic part in play. He elaborates on the *cleavage* between the two and argues that "contact with reality is never entirely lost, the phenomena which we are accustomed to associate with the neuroses are never absent" (Bion, 1957, p. 46). He goes on to say, "On this fact, that the ego retains contact with reality, depends on the existence of a non-psychotic personality parallel with, but obscured by, the psychotic personality" (ibid.).

He then makes a statement that has a profound theoretical and clinical implication:

> The sadistic attacks on the ego and on the matrix of thought, together with projective identification of the fragments make it certain that from this point there is *an ever-widening divergence* between the psychotic and non-psychotic parts of the personality until at last the gulf between them is felt to be *unbridgeable.*
>
> (p. 51, italics added)

Bion then goes on to propose a psychoanalytic theory that is interested in studying the links in the matrix of the psychotic and non-psychotic parts of the mind. He moves away from the dichotomous, binary, disease model and proposes a novel approach in working with patients. The seeds of his container–contained model, which he develops in *Learning from Experience* and "Catastrophic Change", are planted – the psychotic and the non-psychotic trade the function of the container or contained.

Bion's theory is what Arnaldo Chuster (2014, p. 41) calls a spectrum model; there is a spectrum of possibilities in the matrix of the psychotic and non-psychotic parts of the mind. The portion of the electromagnetic spectrum that is visible to the human eye is very limited. There are infra and ultra wavelengths that need a different instrument for observation. In "Making the Best of a Bad Job", Bion (1987a) writes:

> Suppose we respect equally both states of mind, or many states of mind whatever they are: then what state of mind shall we choose for interpretation? Verbal action? That is an everyday problem. In our present culture it is not thought correct to make a rhapsodic response, an immediate abandonment of the screen between impulse and action, translating the impulse direct into action without any intervening delay. It is considered to be equally incorrect to prolong thought to the point at which the action is so delayed that it either does not take place at all, or thinking becomes a substitute for action. When virtually instantaneous action is called for, it is likely to precipitate a response that is rhapsodic, impulse direct to action without any intervention of thought.
>
> (p. 255)

To shine a light on the clinical and technical implications of his newfound theory, Bion shifts the focus of the paper to the importance of symbol formation for the development of verbal thought in the depressive position. For the psychotic part of the mind, he writes "I am concerned with an earlier stage in the same story" (p. 49). He returns to Freud's 1911 paper and highlights two key points. The first is Freud's statement that thought is a function that facilitates the restraint of *action*. The second, Freud's proposition that

> It is probable that thinking was originally unconscious, in so far as it rose above mere ideation and turned to the relations between *object impressions*, and it became endowed with further qualities which were perceptible to consciousness only through its connection with the memory traces of words [italics added].

Bion indicates that the earliest thought is visual, not auditory, and the memory traces of it are perceptible through ideographs. He goes on to infer that, at the preverbal level, *ideograph* is "bound up with awareness of psychic reality" (p. 49).

When the psychotic part of the mind attacks the *links* that makes him aware of the external and internal reality, it is attacking the *link* between *ideographs* and the emotional experience of them. Verbal thought is the result of the synthesis that leads to the communication and articulations of awareness of psychic and external reality. Contained in the matrix are the *links* between one *ideograph* and another. Symbol formation that starts with the conjunction of two objects is deemed difficult, if not impossible, since the psychotic part of the personality has expelled not only the matrix of the *ideographs*, but also the *links* that join them. The psychotic part of the mind, therefore, fails to repair the ego and fails to join the *ideographs* together to "form a new object from which thought springs". *Ideographs*, "spoken but not articulated" (Bion, 1990, p. 13), fail to become a template for verbal thought. On the other hand, the non-psychotic part of the personality introjects the *ideographs* as object impressions, thus providing the matrix with a scaffolding for the development of verbal thought.

Bion (1957, p. 54) suggests that, in the analysis of such patients, the analyst must get in touch with the psychotic part of the patient. He offers a detailed clinical case of a "certifiable psychotic patient". Bion took the patient's response to him, be it in muscular movements or the utterance of disjointed statements, as the patient's mutilated attempt at cooperation, even if the patient rejected his interpretations. A *link*, however thin, was in place. Bion took the movements as a conglomeration of "miniature dramatic presentation", a visual association of the baby's earliest experience – changing diaper, feeding, taking a bath, sexual seduction, and so on. The patient's musculature movements were a means of *expressing* an idea when a verbal representation of it was cut into pieces, or not yet formed – what Bion called ideomotor activities. He associated the ideomotor activity with what Freud attributed to the pleasure principle. The patient's actions were an attempt at the discharge of the accumulation of the undigested stimuli – and not a response to an awareness of the external reality. This clinical experience justified his modifications of Freud's theory of mental functioning. He posited that "the withdrawal from reality is an illusion, not a fact, and arises from the deployment of projective identification against the mental apparatus that was listed by Freud" (p. 46).

In his 1979 paper, Bion made his views explicit: "I would make a distinction between existence – the capacity to exist – and the ambition or aspiration to have an existence which is worth having" (Bion, 1987c, p. 249). A little later in the same paper, he offers a new formula:

> Freud described Two Principles of Mental Functioning; I suggest Three Principles of Living. First, feeling; second, anticipatory thinking; third, feeling plus thinking plus Thinking. The latter is synonymous with prudence or foresight → action.
>
> (p. 255)

Let's look again at the clinical material. In one session the patient says, "[m]y head is splitting; maybe my dark glasses". Bion remembers that, months earlier, he wore dark glasses that seemingly went unnoticed by the patient. Bion heard the patient's comment as a "flash of [his]intuition" (Bion, 1957, p. 157). Since the psychotic part of the mind collapses time and space, Bion surmised that his patient accessed, or rather borrowed, the ideographic memory of Bion's dark glasses from the non-psychotic part of his personality. At this point, it was made available for the psychotic side for a quick repair of his damaged ego.

In the commentary, Bion (1967, p. 153) describes the transference phenomena as changing pictorially from "the line without a breadth" to "the plane without depth". The ideograph of the "dark glasses" created a possibility to shift from linearity to a plane that provided a canvas for complex images and patterns, rather than points and lines. Bion then *linked* the ideographs of the dark glasses to the other ideographs that had been there all along, the musculature movements, the ostensibly nonsensical statements. He was able to *see* the *links* of the object impressions. The dark glasses became a selected fact for his imaginative conjecture. He speculated that, perhaps, the dark glasses contained several meanings. Darkness and glasses, separate and together, provided additional clues to help him unpack the agglomerated bizarre objects. From the matrix of ideographs, he imagined the vestiges of the patient's earliest experiences in infancy. When he made interpretations from this vertex, the plane of the transference turned deeper. Bion observed a significant shift in the patient. The patient's demeanor softened. Bion reported that "at the beginning and end of sessions he met my eyes and did not either evade me or, what with him had been a common event, focus beyond me as if I were the surface of a mirror" (Bion, 1957, p. 60). The onset of time and space in the transference gave rise to depressive feelings and awareness of his utter dependence on his analyst and his objects. When the patient said, "The week-end; don't know if I can last it", Bion made a moving interpretation:

> You feel that you have to be able to get on without me. But to do that you feel you need to be able to *see* what happens around you, and even to be able to contact me; to be able to contact me at a *distance,* as you do your mother when you ring her up; so you tried to get your ability to *see* and *talk* back again from me.
>
> (p. 59; italics added)

Taking the compressed ideographs apart and putting them back together as a new object for introjection made symbol formation and a capacity for self-reflection and mourning possible.

Bion made a brilliant observation that the analyst needs to get in touch with the sane psychotic in himself. Using the psychotic, the scientific, and the religious vertex makes room for the aesthetic dimension and helps the analyst to get in touch with the patient's preverbal, embryonic mind. In the commentary, Bion makes a point to say that a movement from a linear, Euclidean geometry to the planar projective geometry is necessary to access the mind. Movement on a plane is not bidirectional; it is pictorial and allows patterns and phase shifts to emerge. Points and lines, standing for the absent breast and penis, respectively, gain added dimensions and directions in planar projective geometry – a spectrum of possibilities is revealed. In "Making the Best of a Bad Job", Bion writes:

> the analyst needs to be able to listen not only to the words but also to the music, so that he can hear a remark which is not easily translated into black marks on paper, which has a different meaning when it is made in tones of sarcasm, or in terms of affection or understanding.
>
> (Bion, 1979, p. 251)

By the same token, the patterns that emerge in projective geometry, the realization, must be communicated to the patient in terms of the Euclidean space. After all, the analyst's tool of communication is verbal, which is linear, what Arnaldo Chuster refers to as an element in the ethical dimension – contrasted by the aesthetic (Chuster, 2014, p. 118). *Transformation in hallucinosis* is a development of this observation (Bion 1965). Dr. Goldberg and her little patient's interactions are an example of *transformation in hallucinosis*. I also think that Bion's perspective on *intuition* is informed by this capacity to navigate the ethical, verbal, Euclidean elements and the multidimensional aesthetical, nonlinear ones – one informs and transforms the other – there is a container–contained relationship.

Bion takes for granted that *intuition* is inherent in us all. "*It may have occurred to you*, as it often had to me, that I was watching a series of miniature dramatic presentations" (Bion, 1957, p. 54, italics added). Well, I must confess – it did not *occur* to me! But Bion's point is that, to access the psychotic part of the mind, the most vital instrument at the analyst's disposal is his trained intuition, what Jim Grotstein referred to as the analyst's North Star (Chuster, 2020).

In the conclusion of the "Differentiation" paper, Bion (1957) writes

> The patient's destructive attacks on his ego and the substitution of projective identification for repression and introjection must be worked through. Further, I consider that this holds true *for the severe neurotic*, in whom I believe there is a psychotic personality hidden by neurosis as the neurotic personality is screened by psychosis in the psychotic, that has to be laid bare and dealt with.
>
> (p. 63, italics added)

Bion, Klein, and Winnicott each provide a theoretical foundation for working with the psychotic part of "neurotic" patients – patients who, by the way, comprise the bulk of our contemporary clinical practices. Winnicott describes the False Self as that which protects and shields the patient from the storm – the chaos of undigested terror, and the sadness of his True Self. Prognosis, which for Bion means the capacity to traverse the caesura of "psychotic insanity" and "sane psychosis", when seen from a Winnicottian vertex, may depend on the extent to which a link exists between the True and the False Self. From the psychotic and the non-psychotic vertex, prognosis depends on how "wide the divergence" is. This is not to suggest that the True Self is the same as the psychotic, and the False Self, the non-psychotic part. These are just different vertices from which we view the patient's situation. The question is whether the analyst is willing and able to help the patient narrow the gap and introduce the two sides to one another. Two important factors in the analytic function, then, are one mentioned earlier, the analyst's own intuition, and the other, whether the analyst has made the acquaintance of his own psychotic side.

This last point illuminates an issue in training and analyses – something Bion makes a point of in the commentary and in his last paper. In agreement with Melanie Klein's claim that there are psychotic mechanisms in all analysands, he adds that all analysands are fearful of their psychotic side. He gives a vivid illustration of it:

> How awful when you find a maggot in your apple! Not so awful as finding half a maggot in your apple. So, we find that only having half our wits about us is a discovery that is most disturbing. It is one reason why there is a division of opinion as to whether to have all our wits about us, or go back to having only one half – the wakeful, conscious, rational, logical.
>
> (Bion, 1979, p. 254)

So, Bion suggests that the inherent vulnerability of a training analysis is that analytic candidates are human and no different than any other analysand, except they have psychoanalytic training as a refuge. In the commentary, he explicitly wrote about it:

> The individual seeks to deal with his fear by becoming a trainee, so that his acceptance can be taken as an authoritative declaration of immunity by those best qualified to know. He can proceed with the aid of his psychoanalyst to evade coming to grips with his fear and terminate by becoming a pseudo-psychoanalyst. His qualification is an ability, thanks to projective identification (in which he does not believe), to preen himself on freedom from the psychosis for which he looks down upon his patients and colleagues.
>
> (Bion, 1967, p. 162)

Bion appreciates the richness and expanse of the psychotic part of the mind and viewed it as a privilege to work with patients who are psychotic, because it "affords us an opportunity for seeing what it means to work when insane". This sentence can be read in two ways – what Bion termed the reversible perspective: that Bion is talking about the analyst and not just the patient. As Jim Grotstein (2009) once told me, Bion proudly referred to himself as a sane psychotic.

I venture to say that training analysis, no matter how skillfully conducted, does not free one from the pseudo-psychoanalyst. There is a distaste for half a maggot, and having half "our wits" may be the price to pay. However, if the consciousness of the divergence is attended to, "flashes" of having 'our wits about us' may reveal themselves in the consulting room – even in a training analysis. Returning to Freud, the self-analysis that endures lifelong may be a key to minding the gap.

My experience of *forgetting and rereading* this paper revealed the traces of late Bion in his early papers – his thoughts looking for a thinker. In his later work (Bion, 1987a), Bion quoted the poetry of Donne to discuss the *link* between the senses and consciousness of them:

> Her pure and eloquent blood
> Spoke in her cheeks, and so distinctly wrought
> That one might almost say, her body thought

All through the commentary he critiques the idea of cure, an important difference between the early and late Bion. Cure, he asserts, in the service of the pleasure principle, is a sign of the analyst's memory and desire. Instead, he viewed the role of the psychoanalyst as being to get the patient to communicate with the Self; to help the patient to develop the capacity for a reversible perspective; to get psyche-soma and somato-psychic to communicate better with each other – what I understand to be an example of what Humberto Maturana and Francisco Varela refer to as *autopoiesis* (Maturana & Varela, 1980).

Bion (1979/1987c) wrote two simple sentences in his last paper describing "The Three Principles of Living". They are short – but profound. "Three Principles of Living. First. Feeling; second, anticipatory thinking, third, feeling plus thinking plus Thinking. The latter is synonymous with prudence or foresight ⊠ action" (p. 329). With these words, Bion moved from Freud's Darwinian concept of *natural selection* to what Humberto Maturana calls *natural drifts* (Maturana & Mpodozis, 2000). As mentioned earlier, *here* adaptation is conceived as a constant factor in which organisms and structures change congruently – what Maturana (2000) calls *structural coupling*. Maturana's formulation is analogous to the sometimes-confusing language of Bion's *point* and *line*.

The three principles of living, "first, *feeling*; second, *anticipatory thinking*; third, *feeling plus thinking plus Thinking*": *feeling* – the absent breast, the *point*, the source of vitality; *anticipatory thinking – the penis*, the *line*, the dynamic force that gives direction to the *point*. The congruity of *points* and *lines*, in the projective plane, corresponds with Bion's third principle, *feeling plus thinking plus Thinking – Thinking* (capital T) is prudence in action, stressing the importance of the analyst's repose and patience (Bion, 1979).

Throughout the work of Arnaldo Chuster, we hear the same concepts in a language that is experience near:

> *Prudence*, in *action* or foresight, is an ethical proposition to psychoanalysis – real psychoanalysis is real life. Psychoanalysis must do more than deepen knowledge. Psychoanalysis must help patients improve the mental quality of their lives, which is quite an amazing humanistic vertex.
> (Chuster, 2022)

References

Aguayo, J. (2016). Filling in Freud and Klein's maps of psychotic states of mind: Wilfred Bion's reading of Freud's "Formulations regarding two principles in mental functioning". In G. Legorreta & L.J. Brown (Eds.), *On Freud's "Formulations on the Two Principles of Mental Functioning"* (pp. 19–38). Karnac.

Bion, W.R. (1957). Differentiation of the Psychotic from the Non-Psychotic Personalities. In *Second Thoughts: Selected Papers on Psycho-Analysis* (pp. 43–64). Karnac.

Bion, W.R. (1962). *Learning from Experience*. Karnac.

Bion, W.R. (1963). *Elements of Psychoanalysis*. Heinemann.

Bion, W.R. (1965). *Transformations*. Karnac.

Bion, W.R. (1966, 2014). Vol. 6. *Catastrophic Change* (pp. 19–44). In The Complete Works of W.R. Bion. Routledge.

Bion, W.R. (1967). *Second Thoughts: Selected Papers on Psychoanalysis*. Karnac.

Bion, W.R. (1970). *Attention and Interpretation*. Maresfield Library.

Bion, W.R. (1987a). *Clinical Seminars and Other Works*. Fleetwood Press.

Bion, W.R. (19761987b). Evidence. In *Clinical Seminars and Other Works* (pp. 239–246). Fleetwood Press.

Bion, W.R. (1979/1987c). Making the Best of a Bad Job. In *Clinical Seminars and Other Works* (pp. 247–256). Fleetwood Press.

Bion, W.R. (1990). *Brazilian Lectures: 1973 São Paulo 1974 Rio de Janeiro/São Paulo*. Karnac.

Chuster, A. (2014). *A Lonesome Road*. Trio Studio.

Chuster, A. (2020). Personal communication.

Chuster, A. (2022). Personal communication.

Freud, S. (1911). Formulations on the Two Principles of Mental Functioning. In *The Standard Edition of the Complete Psychological Work of Sigmund Freud*. Vol. 12, pp. 213–226. Hogarth.

Freud, S. (1924). Neurosis and Psychosis. In *The Standard Edition of the Complete Psychological Work of Sigmund Freud*. Vol. 19: pp. 147–154. Hogarth.

Grotstein, J. (2009). Personal communication.

Klein, M. (1946). Notes on Some Schizoid Mechanisms. *The International Journal of Psychoanalysis*, 27, 99–110.

Maturana, H. (2000). The Nature of the Laws of Nature. *Systems Research and Behavioral Science*, 17, 459–468.

Maturana, H., & Mpodozis, J. (2000). The Origin of Species by Means of Natural Drift. *Revista Chilena de Historia Natural*, 73(2), 261–310. doi:10.4067/s0716-078x2000000200005

Maturana, H.R. (1999). The Organization of the Living: A Theory of the Living Organization. *International Journal of Human-Computer Studies*, 51(2), 149–168. doi:10.1006/ijhc.1974.0304

Maturana, H.R., & Varela, F.J. (1980). *Autopoiesis and Cognition*. D. Reidel.

Chapter 5

The Limitations of Language in the Psychic Realm[1]

Annie Reiner

In a clinical seminar I attended with Bion (1977), he asked the group, "What language is this patient speaking?" This enigmatic question was like a Zen koan which cannot be answered logically. We can't fall back on what we already understand because it doesn't make any sense, and so it forced us into a different, intuitive mode of thinking. Well, I guess one could answer it logically, "This patient is speaking English, or Spanish, French, and so on," but obviously that is not what he meant. Bion was talking about each person's own idiosyncratic language, reflecting his or her own particular state of mind. He was calling attention to the vagaries of a language created for the *physical* world of the senses, but which analysts have to apply to the *metaphysical* world of the mind—to feelings, thoughts, ideas that have no physical attributes. Feelings cannot be seen, touched, smelled, and so on, and yet we must find a way to talk to people about the nuances of these ephemeral states.

Bion has a reputation for being enigmatic, mysterious, complex, and confusing. I found him at times to be all of those things, but at the same time his vision often derived from the simplest of perceptions, including how we speak and use language. He was essentially questioning the tools of our trade, which, he suggested, may not be up to the job, as I read in the epigram Bion wrote, speaking about our communications with psychoanalytic colleagues:

> [W]e often talk in a way which sounds exactly as if we talked the same language. It is very doubtful.
>
> (Bion, 1975, p. 23)

And here I am, talking to you, not really knowing if we are speaking the same language. But Bion wasn't just being pessimistic; he was trying to find a better way. As for the obstacles in communicating with patients, Bion (1977) often asked, "How can we get the interpretation to the right address?" Are we actually being heard by the patient? As analysts, such as Ferenczi, Klein, Bion, Tustin, and others, began addressing increasingly primitive mental states, we needed a language that could speak to deeper levels of the mind, before or beyond words. These obstacles to being understood are not always

DOI: 10.4324/9781032661230-6

evident to us as analysts, or the analysand, but they are significant, which is why I decided to discuss Bion's ideas about language today.

Everyone Can Talk

Since virtually everyone can talk, we assume we can do so effectively. It may indeed be effective in dealing with everyday life. Mel Brooks, being interviewed as the "2000 Year Old Man," was asked, "What was the first language of cave men?" And Mel replied, "Rock talk. We'd say, 'Put down that rock! Don't throw that rock at me! What are you doing with that rock?!'" (language of concrete objects). But, as Bion pointed out, the language of psychoanalysis, of *inner* life, differs from everyday language based on physical realities, and yet we have to use the same fundamental language for both. As Bion (1992) said, "The language of ordinary human beings is only appropriate to the rational" (p. 371). If we're talking about the metaphysical reality of the mind, such as O, ineffable aspects of mental life, it requires a different language. Grotstein (2007) similarly said, "ordinary (sense-based) language is unsuitable for use in psychoanalysis" (p. 111).

How is it that we haven't noticed this? On the other hand, you may feel I am going on about something that doesn't even seem like an issue. But Bion's early theories of thinking, which are less controversial than his later concept of O, basically redefined what we mean by a "mind." Grotstein and Meltzer (2009) talk about how both Freud and Klein assumed the existence of a mind, able to think about and respond to what we say, but Bion's idea of a mind is of a mental *potential* that either develops in the infant's relationship to the mother or it does not. It led Bion to think that we may also have neglected to ask ourselves whether the human mind—the very focus of our work—exists at all.

> Let us hope that such a thing as a mind, a personality, a character exists, and that we are not just talking about nothing.
>
> (Bion, 2005, p. 317)

Bion never shied away from these fundamental questions, and this one gives voice to the mystery at the heart of psychoanalytic inquiry, namely a mind/self/ personality whose existence is unprovable through sensory means. Bion himself did believe in the existence of this enigmatic mind, but he did not think it was something analysts had agreed upon. It very much relates to the controversy about O, for this unknowable, unprovable mind *is* what Bion called O, the enigmatic realm, which some analysts find ridiculous and believe is unscientific. For Bion, however, it meant we would need a new science able to encompass psychoanalytic knowledge of the mind, and O was his attempt to do so. Contact with O, he said, requires of the analyst, "a peculiar state of mind … [where] the margin between being consciously awake … and being asleep, is extremely small" (Bion, 1978, p. 41) (cf. negative capability). So, what kind of language does that demand us to speak? It is a language some-where between dreaming and waking life.

Clinical Considerations

How is one to detect in the analysand, or the analyst, the presence or absence of a sentient, creative mind, as opposed to a more ego-driven, computer-like artificial intelligence that can absorb and retain data, theories, memories, but cannot feel or think? Patients may appear to hear us, even agree with our interpretations, but we may notice that, at times, they seem unmoved or detached, or that nothing changes. On some level, this might be said to reflect resistance or envy, or negative therapeutic reactions to painful change, but, at a deeper level, it may mean that the patient has not yet developed a mind or self that is truly present. So, here is the analyst, half awake and half asleep, while the patient may be totally asleep, and so unreachable.

One brief example of this is a patient who came in one day complaining that he had trouble sleeping. He woke up multiple times at night and couldn't get back to sleep. He talked about some things that were causing anxiety and he lamented, "I used to be such a good sleeper." He spoke about other things, rage at his boss (and rage was a central issue for him), a problem with his girlfriend, but one sentence continued to reverberate in my ears—"I used to be such a good sleeper." This, I think, was the selected fact, and I said, "You used to be such a good sleeper and then you came here and woke up." What had awakened in the last four years were feelings other than rage—sadness, deep abandonment—vulnerable feelings that used to be instantly killed off by rage. However, not yet knowing quite what to do with these new feelings, he was nostalgic for the good old days when he was sound asleep. "Such a good sleeper."

In supervision, analysts have asked me, what do you mean that the patient has no mind or self? These are aspects of a self, feelings that are hidden, asleep, or unborn. I think it's familiar to us in Winnicott's distinction between the True Self and False Self, whereby problems in the emotional environment (the mother's depression, anxiety, neglect, etc.) can obstruct the development of the infant's authentic self, which is then replaced by a False Self. The individual's entire self may then be a lie, for, "Only the True Self can feel real" (Winnicott, 1965, p. 148). I would say that the False Self is an undeveloped or distorted self, or a non-self, a mind or self whose potential has not developed or awakened. Winnicott (1965) also describes the "fear of breakdown" as a breakdown that occurred in the patient's infancy but cannot be remembered because, "this thing of the past has not happened yet because the patient was not there for it to happen to" (p. 105). The self or mind, that is, was unborn and remains unborn, with no mind to receive or experience the meaning of our interpretations.

Apropos of taking language for granted, Ferenczi (1988) much earlier said, "We talk about the splitting of the personality but do not seem sufficiently to appreciate the depth of these splits" (p. 199). The word, then, does not adequately reflect the actual experience. But how does one speak to split, splintered, or "atomised" bits of a self, a predicament similar to Bion's (1977) question about how to get the interpretation to "the right address." These ideas are not new: they are also seen in Tustin's (1990) writings about autistic states in adults, but what may be different is how prevalent they are in "normal" neurotic states. The question is, who are we talking to? Are we talking to anyone?

Transcendent Truths and Unconscious Lies

What kind of language can traverse the obstacle of an unborn, undeveloped, or non-self? One needs to become a sort of midwife for that unborn self and, basically, to distinguish truth from lies. This sounds simple enough, but these are mental lies that even the individual him- or herself does not know are lies. But people can be dominated by these unconscious "lies," and so the analyst may be talking to a *physically* present patient who does not *psychically* exist.

Another brief example, a sensitive, intuitive, and high-functioning patient whose mother was psychotic. He often boasted of having "a high tolerance for pain." One would certainly need this with a psychotic mother, but it soon became clear to me that this patient had *no* tolerance for pain, having simply killed off all of his painful feelings and his mind. This was not obvious to me, or to him, for he appeared to feel a lot, but, as Ferenczi suggested, the split was so great that his true, as yet unborn, self felt nothing. While, physically, there was nothing wrong with his hearing, he often could not hear or absorb what I said.

The language of an absent or unborn self differs significantly from the language of an authentic self that can feel and think. This is essentially the distinction Bion (1970) makes between the "language of achievement" and the "language of substitution." I won't go into this here, but, briefly, the language of achievement can express psychical states, while the language of substitution is described by Bion (2005) as a "debased currency, words which are worn absolutely smooth till they are meaningless" (p. 315). Among these he includes the often theoretical language of psychoanalysis, advising instead that each analyst "has to [forge] his own language" (ibid.).

I think this clinical vignette illustrates some of these ideas about language.

Clinical Vignette

"Mrs. C" is a bright, successful businesswoman. She was deeply scarred by a needy, depressed mother by whom she constantly felt abandoned and unseen. To give one telling example, the family jokes about forgetting to bring her in from the car when they brought her home from the hospital. About three years into her analysis, Mrs. C described dreams in which, "I keep trying to find solutions to problems that don't exist."

"I dreamt I was at work, re-calculating budgets, endless calculations. I worked hard all night long. When I woke up I thought, 'These aren't real problems … none of this is real.'"

I think this is a good description of the activities, and the language, of an absent self. I suggested to Mrs. C that, despite her tireless calculations, she can't tell what anything is worth, including herself. As a child, her mother's mindlessness made her feel alternately worthless and enraged, but, without a mind to contain and make meaning of these feelings, they went "round and round" within her mind, and still do, for, despite her hard work and determination, she has no way of knowing what is happening inside her. We have come to refer to this as "being on the hamster wheel"—thoughts that go nowhere, moving endlessly back and forth between feelings of being worthless and rage at her mother's worthlessness, then back again to her own guilt and worthlessness for hating her mother.

Mrs. C's endless budgetary computations cannot solve the emotional question of her value to her mother and, ultimately, her right to exist. As this began to be real to her, she became anxious about dying, which always seems to accompany a mental birth. It was a good sign, because one cannot fear death if one is already mentally dead or absent. This was the seed of a mind in her as some feelings came to life. The first "address" I had to find for Mrs. C was her *non*-address, the place where she did not exist, where her feelings were dead. As this absence became painfully real, we began creating a language that had meaning to us both.

The Selected Fact

I want to talk a bit about the "selected fact," one of Bion's (1962) most important and innovative clinical ideas. Given its centrality in his view of psychoanalytic practice, it seems odd how infrequently it is discussed, used, or taught in psychoanalytic institutes, including mine (the Psychoanalytic Center of California). The selected fact addresses the analyst's challenge of how to make sense of the often overwhelming amount of stimuli in a session, to find the relevant fact within the patient's words, feelings, associations, body language, dreams, and so on, and one's own thoughts, reflections, feelings, and so on. (I've written about some of this in my new book, *Bion's Theories of Mind: A Contemporary Introduction*, 2023.)

Bion borrowed the term, "selected fact," from French mathematician Henri Poincaré, who reflected on the difficulties in creating new mathematical formulae.

[A new result] must unite elements long since known, but till then scattered and seemingly foreign to each other, [that] suddenly introduce order where the appearance of disorder reigned … it enables us to see at a glance each of these elements in the place it occupies in the whole.

(Quoted by Bion, 1962, p. 72)

Einstein's $E = mc^2$, for instance, is a distillation of the universe of energy and matter into a simple equation. Much as the mathematician gleans relevant facts from a plethora of scientific data, the analyst must winnow out the relevant idea that gives coherence to the flood of seemingly foreign elements in a session. The selected fact implies the existence of a hidden but fundamental order that, once discovered, introduces unity into the apparent disorder, which serves as the basis of more cohesive and specific interpretation. According to Poincaré, *without* this harmonizing element, the complexity of the world would overwhelm the mind.

The only facts worthy of our attention are those which introduce order into this complexity and so make it accessible to us.

(Bion, 1962, p. 72)

How, though, to determine which facts are or are not relevant? This is a familiar challenge for any psychoanalyst working toward finding the essential meaning in the verbal, emotional, physical, and metaphysical diversity of a session. Like the adage "You can't see the forest for the trees," the organizing principle is right in front of us, but obscured by all the separate parts. One cannot get hung up on the minutiae. Finding the selected fact is like finding a needle in a haystack, a difficult mental task that I think really depends on Bion's (1967a, 1970) later clinical directive to suspend memory, desire, and understanding in order to facilitate contact with O.

When he first spoke of the selected fact in 1962, Bion may not yet have had the language, or understanding, to describe the arcane, enigmatic state of mind of O, but his belief that it was possible to ferret out the essential truth of a session—the selected fact—indicates that he *was* able to conceive of that kind of laser-sharp insight into hidden patterns of the mind. From this perspective, I would view O as a thought without a thinker that eventually found, in Bion, a thinker to think it. Discovering that elusive "needle in an analytic haystack" depends on the deeply intuitive state of suspending memory, desire, understanding—the waking-dream state of O. This kind of surrender of one's mind was like the state described by a 14th-century Christian mystic as "a cloud of unknowing" (Anon., 2020). In that dreamlike cloud, the answer, the selected fact, may cut through the fog like a beacon.

Bion insisted that he was not a mystic, but he also defined access to O as the domain of the "genius" or "exceptional person" (p. 74), removing it from a strictly traditional religious perspective. I think O, in a sense, was the silent partner in Bion's personality that fueled the prolific creativity and fertile imagination that, whatever you call it, his colleagues and students early on recognized as genius.

Clinical Implications

The waking dream state of O, like the mystic's cloud of unknowing, is a suspension of intellectual knowing to facilitate access to intuitive truth. It allows one to hear, as in a poem, that which is written between the lines. Like O, it is impossible to describe how one intuits the organizing function of the selected fact in the seemingly random ephemeral moments in a session. In my experience, it is sometimes a sense of something out of the ordinary, something striking, or striking by its absence, a discrepancy that gives one pause, alerting or focusing one's attention by piercing that dreamlike "cloud of unknowing." It may feel like a special message, almost like a pulsar emitting radio waves, something different or odd, or ordinary. By ridding one's mind of expectations, or theories, a word or phrase, or a mental image or pun, may come to awareness and awaken a different kind of consciousness. Once one is alerted to it, it still may take a while to get its meaning and the coherence it provides amidst otherwise disorderly ramblings.

It is often believed that the mystical state O, of suppressing memory and desire, is meant to yield some extraordinary mystical idea. Bion, on the contrary, said:

> I found that I could experience a flash of the obvious, one is usually so busy looking for something out of the ordinary that one ignores the obvious as if it were of no importance.
>
> (Bion, 1974, p. 103)

Clinical Example

"Stella" is a 42-year-old professional whose mother was narcissistic and emotionally distant, and whose father was bipolar. Stella struggled all her life with states of withdrawal and dissociation and had great difficulty maintaining relationships. For years, any emotional contact with me frightened and humiliated her, and any feelings of gratitude or connection were followed by hostile detachment. Stella recently married a man she respects, but struggles with these ongoing difficulties with intimacy.

Stella felt gratitude toward me in our last session, but began today's session with a deadly silence, some aimless blather, and more silence. I felt suffocated. She then chatted about having been vaccinated for COVID-19 and feeling somewhat guilty since some older people still had not been able to be vaccinated. (Vaccines were new, and scarce, at this point.) She announced, without concern, her disinterest in intercourse with her husband, but had been flirting with a man at her yoga class, behavior that used to excite her, but no longer does.

> I dreamt about Andy, my friend, at work. He told me he refused to get vaccinated and I immediately lost respect for him, I knew I could no longer be his friend.

"I can't understand these anti-vax people," she said, "this is a deadly virus! I also lose respect for people who voted for Trump." She clarified that Andy, whom she likes and respects, did not refuse to be vaccinated in real life and would not vote for Trump.

I found myself feeling confused about Stella's dream. I shared her belief that people need to get vaccinated, but wondered why she made Andy into someone who would not. My mind drifted back to her deadly silence at the beginning of the session, and her detached rambling that made me feel choked, and I suddenly thought that, in her dream, the deadly "virus" against which Stella had been vaccinated was not COVID-19, but "sexuality"—not just genital intercourse but emotional intercourse, psychical and psychoanalytic intercourse, any kind of connection. Unlike Andy, who had refused the vaccination, she was long ago "inoculated" against connection and love, against life, all things from which she is severely split off. This was the selected fact.

Bion (1967b) called the selected fact, "the coming together, by a sudden precipitating intuition, of a mass of apparently unrelated incoherent phenomena which are thereby given coherence and meaning not previously possessed" (p. 127). This mode of thinking is antithetical to what Bion called "forc[ing] a theory to fit a realization" (Bion, 1967b, p. 127). In a way, the selected fact, hidden within the excess of data in a session, is one version of a thought without a thinker, not yet accessible to thought, that must be apprehended intuitively.

This selected fact did bring coherence to all aspects of the session. Her unconcerned disinterest in intercourse with her husband was evidence of this "inoculation" against contact, and I interpreted that Andy represented me—her "work friend" whom she respects on the one hand, but also feels I am foolish enough to have refused being vaccinated against life, sex, and connection, since I keep bothering her about these things. As a result, she wants nothing more to do with me, hence the deadly silence and meaningless prattle at the beginning of the session, communications that were largely anti-communication, anti-contact. Even mentioning her guilt at jumping the line to get vaccinated in real life made sense in this context, for I think it reflected her slowly growing interest in connection with me and the growing awareness of how damaging this emotional "vaccine" has been in her life and to our work.

If I had been thinking logically, I would have missed the point. We all have our personal opinions, and, given my own views, I agreed with Stella that *not* getting vaccinated was foolhardy. However, the language and apparent logic of the dream essentially had to be turned upside down in order to hear the relevant thought. This is the answer to Bion's question, "What language is this patient speaking?"—and it is not the language of logic. My irrelevant political belief that people should be vaccinated was an obstacle to intuiting the real meaning of Stella's communication.

Given her early maternal abandonment, Stella's inoculation against contact is understandable, but it is now an oppressive edict of a deadly, primitive superego promising unconscious protection from the pain of that unavailable mother. As the wall against contact becomes more permeable, she is in a better position to decide which she prefers. At this point, she isn't sure, but seeing Stella's devotion to this emotional "vaccine" gave us both a clearer view of the power of her prohibition against life and the serious obstacle it poses in our work.

Clinical Vignette

I'll say briefly that "Rachel" is an extremely sensitive person who had a lot of early trauma, premature birth, and a violent father. For the first 10 minutes of this session, I had trouble concentrating on what Rachel was saying. This is unusual for me, and I knew something was happening that I did not understand. She told me this dream.

> I was driving my car and realized I couldn't control the brakes. I was completely terrified that I would crash. But suddenly the brakes were okay and it was alright. I was so relieved.

She said a lot more, talking about her new car, the first really good car that she bought for herself. She mentioned a terrifying incident while biking down a hill, thinking the brakes had gone out, and then spoke of her mother's disregard for her feelings, a torment for Rachel since infancy. None of this seemed to fit the relief at the end of her dream. It was still hard for me to concentrate, and, after a long time, I suddenly sensed that instead of her "brakes," this dream had to do with Rachel's "breaks." Once I thought this, everything fell into place, for I could see that the positive outcome in the dream was actually negative. Careening into feelings of terror and helplessness with no brakes, feeling out of control, Rachel's terror simply *breaks* her mind. From this perspective, saying that "suddenly the brakes were okay," means that, once her mind "breaks" and is splintered, everything is okay, for she can no longer feel the terror or helplessness. In fact, there is no longer a mind or self able to feel anything, including the fear that she is now fragmented. My confused, detached, sleepy feeling as she spoke today reflected this flood of unfelt feelings, for I had absorbed the unconscious fragmentation, the utter absence of a mind or anything able to contain what she felt, nothing made sense.

The selected fact here is the idea that these "breaks" were okay, but, by dreaming of this otherwise hidden reality of her breakdown that had been neutralized and turned good, we could begin to see the obstacle to her getting better. What felt to me like mindlessness felt to her like a relief, experiencing her brokenness as everything being "okay." She had embraced those "breaks" from early on and continues to rely on that dissociated state to find relief from the feelings she has never dared to feel.

Summary

Bion (1975) wrote, "In psychoanalysis we have to manufacture our means of communication while we are communicating" (p. 39). The language of psycho-analysis is born of the moment, in our relationship to that particular patient on that particular day. These improvised communications have no shelf life, and trying, as I have today, to communicate *about* what happens in these inter-changes of invisible inner life is impressionistic at best. What actually happens in a session can be known only to the two parties involved, and even for them it is the stuff of dreams. "You had to be there," as the saying goes, but, if one is authentically there, something powerful can transpire, and, despite our inability to capture it fully in language, those who live it can share its benefits.

In describing how these selections are made, Poincaré (1914) said, "Scien-tists believe that there is a hierarchy of facts, and that a judicious selection can be made" (p. 16). Just as scientists talk about the beauty of a theory or equation, based on its simplicity, Poincaré wrote,

> It is the search for this sense of special beauty, the sense of the harmony of the world, that makes us select the facts best suited to contribute to this harmony. ... Thus we see that care for the beautiful leads us to the same selection as care for the useful.
>
> (pp. 22–23)

This scientific statement by Poincaré is very much what Keats said in his famous lines from "Ode on a Grecian Urn."

> "Beauty is truth, truth beauty"—that is all
> Ye know on earth, and all ye need to know.

Another reason to look for the harmony in the session is that it also reflects the harmony in the minds of the patients who dream these dreams. Hearing the selected fact depends upon the capacity for the intuitive waking dream state of Bion's unknowable O. This begins with our having the faith and courage to face our own ignorance, to stop thinking about what we *know* so we can focus on learning what we *don't* know.

Note

1 Some of these ideas first appeared in Reiner (2021) or were written for Reiner (2023).

References

Anonymous. (2020). *The Cloud of Unknowing*. Edited by C. Patel. Las Vegas, NV: Lamplight.

Bion, W.R. (1962). *Learning from Experience*. New York: Basic Books.

Bion, W.R. (1967a). Notes on memory and desire. *Psychoanalytic Forum* 11:3, 271–280.

Bion, W.R. (1967b). The imaginary twin. In *Second Thoughts* (pp. 3–22). New York: Jason Aronson.

Bion, W.R. (1970). *Attention and Interpretation*. London: Basic Books.

Bion, W.R. (1974). *Bion's Brazilian Lectures I: Sao Paulo, 1973*. Rio de Janeiro, Brazil: Imago Editora.

Bion, W.R. (1975). *Bion's Brazilian Lectures II: Rio/Sao Paulo, 1974*. Rio de Janeiro, Brazil: Imago Editora.

Bion, W.R. (1978). *Four Discussion with W. R. Bion*. Perthshire, Scotland: Cluny Press.

Bion, W.R. (1992). *Cogitations*. London: Karnac.

Bion, W.R. (2005). Evidence. In: F. Bion (Ed.), *W.R. Bion, Clinical Seminars and Other Works* (pp. 312–320). London: Karnac.

Bion, W.R. (1977). Clinical seminar, Bion's home, Homewood Road, Los Angeles.

Ferenczi, S. (1988). *The Clinical Diary of Sandor Ferenczi*. Edited by J. Dupont. Cambridge, MA: Harvard University Press.

Grotstein, J. (2007). *A Beam of Intense Darkness*. London: Karnac.

Meltzer, D. (2009). *Studies in Extended Metapsychology. Clinical Application of Bion's Ideas*. London: Karnac.

Reiner, A. (2021). What language are we speaking? Bion and early emotional life. *The American Journal of Psychoanalysis* 81:1, 6–26.

Reiner, A. (2023). *W.R. Bion's Theories of Mind: A Contemporary Introduction*. London: Routledge.

Tustin, F. (1990). *The Protective Shell in Children and Adults*. London, New York: Karnac.

Winnicott, D.W. (1965). Ego distortions in terms of True and False Self. In *The Maturational Process and the Facilitating Environment* (pp. 140–152). London: Karnac.

Chapter 6

The Clinical Importance of Frustration

Nicola Abel-Hirsch

In Bion's later work there is less general discussion of frustration, but its significance is ever-present clinically. I give examples from a Brazilian supervision and from his dispute with Greenson about the appropriateness – or not – of exposing patients to frustration by not being immediately responsive to their preexisting way of being.

André Green, in his review of Bion's *Cogitations*, comments that:

> It was in October 1959 that Bion had the intuition of the theoretical importance of frustration. [He] must take the credit for the cardinal distinction between frustration evasion and frustration modification. ... Bion made this distinction the foundation of his system.
>
> (Green 1992, p. 586)

I am going to begin with Bion's 'Theory of Thinking' paper, given to the IPA Congress in Edinburgh in 1962 and published in the *International Journal of Psychoanalysis* in the same year. It presents Bion's model of the mind, and, at the heart of his model, he puts a person's relation to the experience of frustration. Bion identifies three broad relations a person can have to frustration:

1 The evasion of frustration. If the evasion of frustration is extreme, a person will attack his or her own mind and contact with reality to evade the cause of the frustration.
2 At the other end of the continuum, we have the healthy suffering and modification of frustration.
3 In the middle of the continuum is where many of our patients frequently are (and where we can be too). Frustration is not evaded to the degree that results in psychosis. Neither is it modified enough for an accurate, durable relation to internal and external reality. Instead, the person is only able to function overly dominated by omnipotence, omniscience and moralistic judgement.

DOI: 10.4324/9781032661230-7

I am going to begin with quotes from the 'Theory of Thinking' paper and then talk briefly about a patient – someone who is dominated by omnipotence, omniscience and moralistic judgement – and both her and my relation to frustration in the analysis.

I will also look at aspects of Bion's own relation to frustration and then at the clinical significance of frustration in his later work. We will look at a comment he makes in one of his 1970s Brazilian supervisions and his dispute with Greenson in Los Angeles, 1967, about the appropriateness – or not – of exposing a patient to frustration.

The terms frustration and impatience may mislead us into thinking this is all about something relatively ordinary. Bion, however, knows personally about the frustration of one's absolute needs that can be felt to imperil the self's viability, including the frustration of his instinct to survive, under the assault of enemy fire and the incompetence of his seniors in World War I. Also, his well-known reference to a mother's impatience with her child's cry may well not be ordinary impatience and may have in it her fear the crying could cause her to feel unbearably helpless. She can't experience the frustration and pushes it back at the infant.

A Theory of Thinking, 1962

The page numbers in this section refer to the Complete Works of W.R. Bion.

> I shall limit the term 'thought' to the mating of a pre-conception with a frustration. The model I propose is that of an infant whose expectation of a breast is mated with a realization of no breast available for satisfaction.
> (Bion, 1962, p. 154)

Bion's container–contained model is one of the development of thought in the presence of the containing parent or analyst. Yet, he says that he is going to limit use of the term 'thought' to the mating of a preconception (expectation of the breast) with a frustration (absence of the breast). Freud talked about how, in the absence of the breast, the infant hallucinates the experience of its presence. You can see this with infants when, in the absence of the breast, they first move their mouths, sucking, until the wait gets too long and they start to cry. In Bion's view, the hungry, distressing experience is first of all experienced as a present bad thing, but then, in health and over time, the infant gradually becomes able to tolerate and experience absence. When the breast is there, we don't need to think. When it is absent, we become able to think in a very rudimentary way that there is a breast, and it's not here. One of the ways in which this is illuminating clinically, and we will see it in relation to my patient, is whether the patient can hold on to a sense of the analytic work at the end of the session and between sessions.

Bion then differentiates between the evasion of the experience of frustration, the experience/modification of the frustration, and the border region between these two. In the border region, the personality rejects the experience of dependence on a breast that is not always present and, instead, fosters the omnipotent/omniscient state of mind in which the self is put in a superior position. The milk is drunk, but without a sense of a psychic/emotional dependent relation to the mother. Bion:

> If intolerance of frustration is not so great as to activate the mechanisms of evasion and yet is too great to bear dominance of the reality principle, the personality develops omnipotence as a substitute for the mating of the pre-conception, or conception, with the negative realization [the mating of knowledge of the breast with the absence of the breast].

Bion goes on:

> This involves the assumption of omniscience as a substitute for learning from experience by aid of thoughts and thinking. There is therefore no psychic activity to discriminate between true and false. Omniscience substitutes for the discrimination between true and false a dictatorial affirmation that one thing is morally right and the other wrong.
>
> (Bion 1962, pp. 156–157)

The two quotes bring to mind a patient who, I think, does tend to put herself in a position of moralistic ascendency, in which her feelings are accounted for by the failures of her objects. I saw this initially in relation to her childhood experience of the birth of her brother. She had not known herself to be angry because she didn't want there to be another baby; hers was experienced as justified anger because of the faults of her parents. In the analysis, she had a belief that her distress about separation should not have to happen. A serious consequence of this is that she is left in my absence with a sense not of a reliable analyst who will return, but of a damaged, untrustworthy object of no use to her.

The patient's difficulty with frustration does not show in any overt impulsive behaviour. Quite the opposite: if anything, she is hyper thoughtful. This, however, can be a way of controlling ever being exposed to frustration. She wants to have seen and taken account of everything before it happens.

I am aware with my patient that sometimes I am interpreting her damaged view of me not from a position of thinking, but like a knee-jerk reaction. A reaction to feeling myself to be under threat? So, in a more paranoid schizoid state myself? Writing this paper has raised a question for me about what I may be avoiding feeling at that moment. In the quote above, Bion comments that "There is therefore no psychic activity to discriminate between true and false. Omniscience substitutes for the discrimination between true and false a dictatorial affirmation that one thing is morally right and the other wrong". The patient and I are vulnerable to deteriorating into a battle about which of us is doing something morally bad, which of us is to blame. The "dictatorial affirmation that one thing is morally right and the other wrong" being itself in these moments indicative of a loss of psychic activity.

So What About Frustration in the Analyst? What About Bion's Own Experiences of Frustration?

There is quite a lot in his autobiography, *The Long Weekend* (1982), about the sexual frustration of adolescence.

We see in his writings on World War I the profound and terrible frustration of his instinct to survive, under the assault of enemy fire and the incompetence of his seniors. What happened when Bion's own men didn't do what he commanded? One gets the impression that most of the time they did (he had authority, he could be trusted); there is a striking incident, however, when they didn't, when newly arrived Welsh coal miners refused to come out of their huts and parade. The incident occurred after the Armistice.

> 'Sir!' saluted Sergeant Major Cannon, 'Company refuses to come on parade.' 'Tell them not to be so bloody silly' [responds Bion]. Off he went. Here was a fine state of affairs. I had not the remotest idea what to do.
>
> All this stuff about the Guards – devilish awkward if it turned out to be true. Now my own company! I felt I would break out in a sweat at any moment. Suppose they still refused. They were nearly all new men, recently trained miners; they hated the army ...
>
> 'Sir!' ...
>
> 'Yes, Sergeant Major?' 'They won't come out sir.'
>
> I knew it. What do I do now? No idea. It was with surprise and relief that I heard myself say, 'Tell the Lewis gun crews to fall in with their guns at once. Post them to cover the huts.'
>
> 'Sir!' ... He was back again in less than five minutes. 'They are in position sir. Six guns facing the huts.'
>
> 'With the hill behind the huts?'
>
> 'Yes sir.'

The Armistice had been signed, but the order was to remain on battle-alert terms. Bion himself comments elsewhere that, if the army were to stand down, it would be almost impossible to get it going again. The newly arrived Welsh miners were refusing to parade in various companies along the line, not only Bion's. I don't know what happened in the other places, but Bion has the guns turned on his company. When he went to inspect the guns, Bion comments, 'I chose not to remark that they were loaded with ball ammunition'. 'Ball ammunition', I discovered, leads to less severe wounding. The gunners believed he might actually order them to fire. After a tense interlude, the Guards emerged to parade.

> Bion: 'Sergeant Major Cannon tells me you fellows didn't want to come on parade. You forget the war's not over – this is only an armistice. We'd have looked a bloody lot of fools if the Boches [Germans] had come over there' – I pointed my stick at the hills behind – 'and caught us while you were all stuck in there.'
>
> (Bion 1982, pp. 315–317)

Bion has had the guns turned to 'cover the huts', 'with the hill behind the huts'. This meant that the guns were turned on the men, but also on the hill behind, from which the Germans could come, against whom Bion wanted himself and the men to be united.

A second example of his response to a frustrating experience, this time from World War II. Bion has arrived at Northfield hospital for soldiers invalided out of the war being fought in Europe.

> Bion: No sooner was I seated before desk and papers than I was beset with urgent problems posed by importunate patients and others. Would I see the NCOs in charge of the training wing and explain to them what their duties were? Would I see Private A who had an urgent need for 48 hours' leave to see an old friend just back from the Middle East? Private B, on the other hand, would seek advice because an unfortunate delay on the railway had laid him open to misunderstanding as one who had overstayed his leave. And so on. ...
>
> Exasperated at what I felt to be a postponement of my work, I turned to consider this problem.
>
> (Bion 1961, pp. 105–106)

Bion is exasperated. I think he then does something rather like turning the guns on the huts with the hill behind. Just as he aimed to unite with the Welsh Guards against the Boche who might come over the hill, he identifies the enemy that is shared by himself and the men at Northfield. The enemy is neurosis.

> Bion: The common danger in the training wing was the existence of neurosis as a disability of the community. ... Neurosis needs to be displayed as a danger to the group; and its display must somehow be made the common aim of the group.
>
> (Bion 1961, pp. 106–107)

As part of his 'displaying' the evidence of neurosis, Bion would walk around the wing and invite men to join him 'just to see how the rest of the world lives' (Bion 1985, p. 110). He encouraged the men's making of informal observations as well as the observations made in the groups and meetings.

In a second incident at Northfield, it is the men who are frustrated. They protest to Bion that only 20% of the men are participating in the new programme, while 80% are shirking. They want Bion to make it stop happening. We might say the men want to evacuate their frustration into Bion. Bion's response is to formulate the 20/80% in Northfield as a particular instance of a general human phenomenon (there are, everywhere, the people who do and the ones who shirk). Bion's intention is to interest the men in the study of the phenomenon they had wanted to get rid of.

Now we fast-forward twenty or so years. Bion is of the view that analysts (including himself) don't realise the extent to which they may be withdrawing from the difficult realities involved in analytic work. In 1968, he writes in a letter to his wife:

> Something was going wrong in the work in England – not only mine. I can't, as you know, pretend I like it, but there it is.
>
> (Bion 1985, pp. 176–177)

The year before, in Los Angeles, he indicated something of what he thought was going wrong:

> I think it is the easiest thing in the world, what with the patients trying to deny the reality of what we are trying to draw attention to, and our own dislike of what we feel we ought to draw attention to, that you can very easily get into a state in which you gradually drift into a position in which you talk not English, but jargon, and in which you talk about the non-existent. It simply becomes a complete myth. Now the serious thing for analysts about this, is that the situation gradually gets more and more intolerable. One is reduced more and more, to denying the reality of something of whose reality we have been at some point absolutely convinced, and which is the one thing that we are really in existence to deal with.
>
> (Bion 2013, pp. 37–38)

Bion's response to what is going wrong is not unlike turning the guns on the huts, with the hills behind, or identifying the enemy of neurosis. He identifies an enemy and aims to interest his colleagues in working with him against the enemy. The enemy now identified is 'memory and desire'. His 1965 paper, 'Notes on Memory and Desire', is unusual in its severely prescriptive tone. In his Introduction in the Complete Works to Bion's 'Notes on Memory and Desire' paper, editor Chris Mawson comments:

> I have written a longer introduction to this paper because of its important place in Bion's thinking and because of the many serious

misunderstandings to which the short and pithy 'Notes on Memory and Desire' has given rise. One such source of misunderstanding is the emphatic and rather uncharacteristically dogmatic tone of parts of the 1965 presentation.

(Bion 1965, p. 4)

I am suggesting that his uncharacteristically prescriptive tone may have a root in his previous military responses to frustrating situations. If correct, it is a sign, I think, of just how frustrated he may have been with what he saw as defensive clinical behaviour – clinical behaviour that lacked both intuitive contact with the patient and the necessary clinical discipline to make this possible. How his reading of the mystical writers St John of the Cross and Meister Eckhart may have changed his more military response to frustration might be something we could discuss.

Bion on the Clinical Significance of Frustration in the late 60s and 70s

We are now getting into Bion's later work. To my knowledge, he doesn't make much further reference to what André Green called the 'theoretical importance of frustration' in his early 60s 'Theory of Thinking' model of the mind. However, his understanding of the significance of frustration is very present in his clinical work. Here is a quote from a later supervision. This is from *Bion in Brazil*, Volume 1 (De Mattos et al. 2017). The book contains previously unpublished supervisions from 1973–1978. My quotes are from Chapter 1, Supervision A1.

In the supervision, we hear that the patient has said to the analyst 'Speak, tell me anything, make even a noise, because I can't stand the silence'.

Bion comments:

> But the statement the patient has made is, in fact, putting pressure on the analyst to make him talk – because if the analyst doesn't talk the patient might go away and never come back again. ... On the other hand, if the analyst does talk, he may be compelled to talk prematurely before he wants to. Now, why can't this patient stand a silence? ...

Bion continues:

> He is both dependent on the analyst being there – which is a nasty feeling – and he is all-alone, which is also a nasty experience. ... If I thought the patient might walk out and leave the room, I think, although I mightn't want to say anything, I would say what I've just said. I would say: 'You are finding this very frightening to be all-alone in this room with me. Perhaps we shall find out, perhaps we shall understand this

more later.' I would prefer, if I could, not to say anymore – but I would prefer, if I could, not to increase the patient's anxiety, either by remaining silent, or by saying too much.

Bion:

> Now, I think that this particular patient also, may not be at all familiar with frustrations, because I suspect, very strongly, that he has learnt to behave like everybody else, in the way that a good mimic can. The sort of mimic, who can professionally take up an acting profession. He isn't good enough to be able to do that. So he's not a professional actor/actress. But he isn't good enough to be real either. So, this matter is difficult, because part of the analytic situation is, for the patient to get used to frustration and it helps him to feel that the analyst, likewise, is frustrated, but is not so frightened of it.

I want to emphasise the last sentence:

> So, this matter is difficult, because part of the analytic situation is, for the patient to get used to frustration and it helps him to feel that the analyst, likewise, is frustrated, but is not so frightened of it.

Brazilian Lecture 7

In his Brazilian Lecture 7 (Bion 1973–1974), Bion makes reference to a mother's impatience – in fact, very probably the mother of the patient in 'On Arrogance' (1958) and further discussed in 'Attacks on Linking' (1959).

> Bion … let us imagine that the baby is very upset and feels afraid of an impending disaster like dying, which it expresses by crying. That kind of language may be both comprehensible and disturbing to the mother who reacts by expressing anxiety – 'I don't know what's the matter with the child!' The infant feels the mother's anxiety and impatience and is compelled to take its own anxiety back again.
> (Bion 1973–1974, 1973 Sao Paulo Lecture, p. 55)

This is the mother who was not able to take in her infant's projections, thinking about whom contributed to Bion's formulation of his concept of the container–contained in 'On Arrogance' onwards. In the Brazilian Lecture some fifteen years later, quoted above, Bion talks about how the infant feels the mothers impatience and anxiety and is compelled to take its own anxiety back. The infant may then become silent and enclose within itself 'a frightening and bad thing'. Something that hasn't found a home in the relationship with the mother. It is this kind of thing that Bion wants to be available to. In his view, communicating his availability to the patient involves not fitting in with the responses the patient might usually elicit, which may involve exposing the patient to frustration. Back in Los Angeles, he had a somewhat heated debate with Greenson about this.

Bion, Greenson and Questions about Exposing Vulnerable Patients to Frustration

Back in 1967 in Los Angeles, Greenson criticised Bion for not being responsive enough to patients and putting them under too much stress.

First Seminar – 12 April 1967

> Greenson ... I think that's very admirable [suppression of memory and desire]. ... [But is it not] a terrible stress on some patients, and shouldn't that be in some way dealt with? I think that with patients who are in analysis for a period of time and can bear this kind of stress, but now what about the patient who isn't in that state?
>
> (Bion 2013, p. 94)

> Greenson: interrupting: No, I want to say I am talking about the danger that you seem to pose by this experiment of creating a situation in which you are dealing with a human being, a unique human being who came to you with problems and a need for help, and now, for some scientific reasons and in order to improve your own insight in time, you're going to put aside his therapeutic needs. You put this into the background, suppress it. You put aside what you know about theory, all of which I can understand temporarily as being a great help in clarifying and freshening your own receptivity to his material. Nevertheless, he's got to leave that hour! And what you do say, 'Good afternoon'?
>
> (Bion 2013, pp. 97–98)

> Bion: ... what I am arguing in favour of is that one should try not to let that pressure [the patient's distress] distort one's judgment. I think that in my experience, the patient can feel something ... about your failure to be jockeyed into a premature interpretation, which gives him something to go on with. Now, this again, is one of these experiences which I think brings it home to you, that we as psychoanalysts are dealing with forces of no mean order, that they are extremely mysterious, they cannot easily be fitted into any form of words (some of them can, but a great many can't), but I think that one can take a certain degree of comfort by that, that actually the inability to give an interpretation (the lack of knowledge about it), and the ability to tolerate the ignorance and the distress of the situation with a

feeling that heaven knows what this patient is going to get up to before he turns up the next day. It self-communicates itself to the patient.

(Bion 2013, pp. 99–100)

Each man thinks that what the other is doing with patients is somewhat dangerous. Greenson sees Bion as unsupportive, Bion thinks that Greenson's responsiveness to the patient may fail to convey that he or she (the analyst) is available to see aspects of the patient that have never had a home. A patient, for example, who as an infant may have become silent and enclosed within itself 'a frightening and bad thing'. Something that hasn't found a home in the relationship with the mother.

Conclusion

I began with quotes from Bion's 1962 'Theory of Thinking' paper. In the first quote, he says he will reserve the term 'thought' for situations in which an expectation is not realised – frustratingly not realised. In the further two quotes, he differentiates between the evasion of frustration, the healthy experiencing of frustration, and a third area, a borderland between the two, in which the person must function under the dominance of omnipotence, omniscience and moralistic judgement.

I gave a clinical example of my work with a patient who, while living a full life, has a part of herself dominated by omnipotence, omniscience and moralistic judgement. I described times when we were both battling in a mire of moralistic judgement about which of us was 'bad' and raised the question of whether, at such times, I was avoiding my own frustration with the work.

Frustration in the analyst: I looked at some ways in which Bion himself responded to frustration and thought I could identify a pattern in which he responded by identifying an enemy and inviting the people he was frustrated with to join him against the enemy. The enemies identified were the Germans in World War I, neurosis in World War II and 'memory and desire' in 1965. I wondered how his reading of the mystics may have contributed to a change in his more military model.

In the last part of the paper, I suggested that what André Green had described as the 'theoretical importance of frustration' in his earlier work was less in evidence in his later work, but that the clinical significance of frustration in his practice was evident. I quoted Bion from a supervision in which he said that 'part of the analytic situation is, for the patient to get used to frustration and it helps him to feel that the analyst, likewise, is frustrated, but is not so frightened of it'. Then I went to his dispute with Greenson in 1967 in Los Angeles. Greenson thought Bion unsupportive of vulnerable patients. Bion thought that responding to the patient in a supportive way can be to enact what was already familiar to the patient and miss the chance of conveying an availability for what might never have found a place in the world.

Bion's identification of the significance of frustration and our different responses to it is well known to many of us theoretically (in relation to his 1962 model of the mind). I suspect there is more to be understood about its significance clinically.

References

Bion, W.R. (1958, 2014). On arrogance. In Vol. 6 (pp. 131–137). The Complete Works of W.R. Bion. Routledge.

Bion, W.R. (1959, 2014). Attacks on linking. In Vol. 6 (pp. 138–152). The Complete Works of W.R. Bion. Routledge.

Bion, W.R. (1961, 2014). Experiences in groups and other papers. In Vol. 4. The Complete Works of W.R. Bion. Routledge.

Bion, W.R. (1962, 2014). The psycho-analytic study of thinking. In Vol. 6 (pp. 153–161). The Complete Works of W.R. Bion. Routledge.

Bion, W.R. (1965, 2014). Memory and desire. In Vol. 6 (pp.1–19). The Complete Works of W.R. Bion. Routledge.

Bion, W.R. (1973–1974, 2014). Brazilian lectures. In Vol. 7 (pp. 1–197). The Complete Works of W.R. Bion. Routledge.

Bion, W.R. (1982, 2014). Vol. 1. *The Long Weekend 1897–1919: Part of a Life* (pp. 13–318). In The Complete Works of W.R. Bion. Routledge.

Bion, W.R. (1985, 2014). Vol. 2. *All My Sins Remembered: Another Part of a Life & The Other Side of Genius: Family Letters.* In The Complete Works of W.R. Bion. Routledge.

Bion, W.R. (2013). *Los Angeles Seminars and Supervision.* Routledge.

De Mattos, Junqueira, de Mattos Brito, Gisele, and Levine, Howard B. (Eds.) (2017). *Bion in Brazil: Supervisions and Commentaries.* London: Karnac.

Green, A. (1992). "Cogitations". By Wilfred R. Bion (Book Review). *International Journal of Psychoanalysis* 73: 585–589.

Chapter 7

Attention and Interpretation

Howard B. Levine

Introduction

Some people who read mystery novels like to begin by looking at the last chapter to find out 'who done it.' If we apply that same principle to Bion's *Attention and Interpretation* (1970), we find in his references at the end of the book one paper by Freud: "On the Two Principles of Mental Functioning." It is there that we will begin. If we read Freud's paper in the light of what Bion wrote about in *Attention and Interpretation*, we can see the Freudian foundation as an important starting point of his thinking.

Freud begins with the statement that

> every neurosis has as its result, and probably therefore as its purpose, a forcing of the patient out of real life, an alienating of him from reality. ... Neurotics turn away from reality because they find it unbearable – either the whole or parts of it.
>
> (1911, p. 218)

In *Attention and Interpretation*, Bion (1970) contrasts the difference between two kinds of patients or states of mind: those who can and those who cannot stand to remain in contact with an anxiety-producing or frustrating reality long enough to tolerate and think about what, if anything, can be done about it, rather than react by trying to evade, deny or distort the perception of the source of their frustration or displeasure.

Bion (1970) writes:

> There are patients whose contact with reality presents most difficulty when that reality is their own mental state ... [P]eople exist who are so intolerant of pain or frustration (or in whom pain or frustration is so intolerable) that they feel the pain but will not suffer it and so cannot be said to discover it. *What* it is that they will not suffer or discover we have to conjecture from what we learn from patients who *do* allow themselves to suffer. The patient who will not suffer pain fails to 'suffer' pleasure and

DOI: 10.4324/9781032661230-8

this denies the patient the encouragement he might otherwise receive from accidental or intrinsic relief.

(p. 9)

Back to Freud (1911)

The pleasure principle leads the individual's mind and psychic activity to strive towards whatever gives pleasure and draw back "from any event which might arouse unpleasure" (p. 219). When "peremptory demands of internal needs ... [disturb the peace of one's resting state,] whatever was thought of (wished for) was simply presented in a hallucinatory manner" (p. 219). This is a summary of his description in *The Interpretation of Dreams* (Freud 1900) of the infant using a perceptual identity (hallucination) of an earlier feed to try to relieve its hunger.

When this fails to relieve its distress, as it inevitably will, "this attempt at satisfaction by means of hallucination" (Freud 1911, p. 219) is abandoned.

> Instead ... the psychical apparatus ... [must decide] to form a conception of the real circumstances in the external world and to endeavor to make a real alteration in them. A new principle of mental functioning [is] thus introduced: what [is] presented in the mind [is] no longer what [is] agreeable but what [is] real, even if it happened to be disagreeable.
>
> (Freud 1911, p. 219)

Thus, Freud describes the setting up of the reality principle.
He goes on:

> The increased significance of external reality heightened the importance of the sense-organs that are directed towards [the] external world, and of the *consciousness* attached to them. Consciousness now learned to comprehend sensory qualities in addition to the qualities of pleasure and unpleasure, which hitherto had been of interest to it. A special function was instituted which had periodically to search the external world, in order that its data might be familiar already if an urgent internal need should arise – [this is] the function of *attention* ... At the same time, probably, a system of *notation* was introduced, whose task it was to lay down the results of this periodical activity of consciousness – a part of what we call *memory*.
>
> (Freud 1911, pp. 220–221; original italics)

Another ego function that must develop in accordance with the need to assess external reality is that of an

> *impartial passing of judgement*, which has to decide whether a given idea was true or false – that is, whether it was in agreement with reality or

not – the decision being determined by making a comparison with the memory-traces of reality. [And,] a new function [is] allotted to motor discharge, which, under the dominance of the pleasure principle, had served as a means of unburdening the mental apparatus of accretions of stimuli. ... Motor discharge was now employed in the appropriate alteration of reality; it [is] converted into *action*.

(Freud 1911, p. 221; original italics)

Freud (1911) adds:

Restraint upon motor discharge (upon action) ... [becomes necessary and is] provided by means of the process of *thinking*, which was developed from the presentation of ideas. Thinking was endowed with characteristics which made it possible for the mental apparatus to tolerate an increased tension of stimulus while the process of discharge was postponed.

(p. 221; original italics)

We see that Freud's formulation of the birth of the capacity for thought is based upon frustration and the absence of the object. The production of thoughts depends upon psychic tension and is a means of regulating and keeping it within optimal, tolerable limits. If this can be done, and frustration can be tolerated, then one can maintain contact with reality and realize one's *truth*. To summarize, the distinction between internal fantasy and external reality will require and depend upon the development and strengthening of the ego functions of attention, notation and the judgment to accurately record, note and assess the truth about what is (external reality).

The Centrality of Frustration Tolerance

For both Freud and Bion, the birth of thought and the capacity to think are dependent upon the ability to tolerate some degree of frustration caused by an absent, ungratifying object. However, it is important to note that, for Freud, or how Freud has been interpreted in regard to neurosis, the gratification at stake revolves around forbidden pleasures. For Bion – and Winnicott[1] – the 'frustration' often concerns the failure of the object or environment to satisfy what Winnicott called "ego needs" needed for the growth, stabilization and coherence of the very sense of self. In these circumstances, 'failure of gratification' refers to what can not just lead to displeasure, but can produce states of 'nameless dread' and other forms of catastrophic annihilation anxiety that threaten the integrity of the self.

With non-neurotic patients and states of mind, keeping the stress of self-disrupting or self-annihilating forces within optimal, tolerable limits is what proves crucial. The experience of the absence of *something*, an object or environmental provision, that is needed but felt to be absent can initiate thoughts – or their precursors, proto-thoughts – or actions. Bion (1962) describes how this desired or needed 'something' is apt to be felt as a "bad object" that must be gotten rid of "either by evacuation or modification. The problem is solved by evacuation if the personality is dominated by the impulse to evade frustration and by thinking the objects if the personality is dominated by the impulse to modify the frustration" (p. 84).

Thus, Bion (1962, 1970) follows Freud (1911) in arguing that thought – and/or the capacity to think thoughts – plays a vital role in, and is dependent upon, frustration tolerance. But, if the frustration related to the actuality of the object – which can take various forms, such as physical absence, mis-attunement, non-receptivity, reversed projective identification, and so on – exceeds whatever the individual's level of 'tolerable' is, then the result will be measures designed to evade frustration by evacuation or the disabling of the means by which one perceives the frustration, rather than recognizing, think-ing about and trying to actually modify the frustrating situation. The impor-tant lesson for the treatment situation is this:

> The choice that matters to the psycho-analyst is one that lies between *procedures designed to evade frustration and those designed to modify it. That is the critical decision.*
>
> (Bion 1962, p. 29, original italics)

Language, Thought and Experience

When seen from the vertex of everyday life and consensually validatable reality, the practice of psychoanalysis, with its attempt to address and impact emotional experience, psychic reality, psychic development and psychic functioning, may appear at times to be counterintuitive, elusive, confusing, even arcane. Despite being a 'talking cure,' there are problems in communication in psychoanalysis that seem almost insurmountable. Some relate to the inherent limitations of language – and perhaps even thought – when attempting to speak or even think about the psyche and emotions. Others have to do with problems of frustration tolerance, the all too human tendency to try to avoid the disturbance often associated with encountering new ideas and the self-deceiving pseudo-omniscience born of intolerance of uncertainty and not knowing.

Any attempt to follow Bion's thinking about these matters immediately plunges the reader into an epistemological conundrum. For Bion (1970), "mental space [i.e., the human psyche] is a thing-in-itself, that is infinite and unknowable, but ... [nevertheless] can be represented by thoughts" (Bion 1970, p. 11).[2] That is, while the fullness of mental 'space' and the phenomena of raw, existential Experience are overwhelmingly infinite, that 'part' of the psyche that contains the set of representations that we speak of colloquially as our 'mind' and its 'thoughts' is three-dimensional.

It is the latter, thoughts, that might come to be known or perhaps only known about. But if so, by what means, and how fully? There is a disparity – and a slippage – as one moves from the thing-in-itself, mental space, raw, existential Experience[3] (O), to what can be known of that experience (K) and again as that knowable part, what we colloquially call 'experience' written with a small e, is spoken of and perhaps too, even as it is thought about.[4] There is an inevitable gap between what is sensuously *felt* and what can be *known* as one moves from the domain of O to that of K. This limitation in *translation*[5] also occurs as one attempts to speak and put the knowable part of our perceptions, thoughts and feelings into words.

From Infinite to Finite: Representation and Transformation

In this gradient or trajectory from raw, existential Experience to not-yet-articulated thought to that portion of thought that can be verbalized, at each point of transition, an unknowable, untransformable residue remains left behind, unrepresented and irrepresentable.[6] This formulation becomes especially relevant as we explore Bion's attempts to expand psychoanalytic theory so as to enable us to "approach a mental life unmapped by the theories elaborated for the understanding of neurosis" (Bion 1970, p. 37).

Neurosis implies psychically *represented* thoughts, wishes and fantasies that are fully saturated in regard to ideational content and are repressed because they are in conflict with the standards and values of one's superego and ego ideal. Ideational contents are repressed and hidden from awareness because of their unacceptability and the anxiety and/or disapproval that they might engender. But, while hidden, these ideational contents remain intact and fully saturated in regard to meaning. The therapeutic goal when addressing the repressed is that of making the unconscious conscious and healing the splits that repression might produce. However, our mental life and what needs to be dealt with in therapy include far more than that which is represented but hidden in the mind.[7]

Bion's (1965, 1970) descriptions of O, beta elements, waking dream thoughts and container–contained all speak to this necessity and indicate processes that contain, transform and metabolize the somato-psychic forces and turbulence of the unrepresented. It is the support, catalysis and co-construction of these movements that lie at the heart of Ferro's (2002) clinical application of Bion's work.

Experience and experience

The disparity between the infinite (mental space) and its representations (thought and that which can be spoken of) is complicated even further by the fact that direct access to or recognition of the fundamental elements of psychoanalytic concern, *emotions* and raw, existential *Experience*, cannot come to be known empirically via the physical senses:

[T]he physician is dependent on realization of sensuous experience in contrast with the psycho-analyst whose dependence is on experience that is not sensuous. The physician can see and touch and smell. The realizations with which a psycho-analyst deals cannot be seen or touched; anxiety has no shape or colour, smell or sound.

(Bion 1970, p. 7)

The situation of the analyst trying to discern the patient's emotions is analogous to that of the physicist trying to observe an atomic particle in a cloud chamber. The particle itself can never be directly observed, but it does announce its presence by leaving a vapor trail in the chamber. So, too, anxiety in the patient. The latter can never be directly 'known' by the analyst, but may 'announce itself' by disrupted speech, rapid breathing, a quickened pulse, the smell of sweat and so on. If that 'knowing' – more likely a hypothesis about its presence – does come about, it does so via *intuition* or conjecture. This raises enormous problems concerning suggestion and compliance, evidence, truth and validation, especially if one's theories of analytic understanding and technique are aligned to content (facts, details, data regarding what is or what happened) rather than process.[8]

Sensuous and Non-Sensuous Experience

In addition to the difficulties in coming to know the very things that psychoanalysts need to speak about, language, because of its inherent nature and the ends to which it can be put, presents its own problems and proves to be an inconstant ally. Bion (1970) begins *Attention and Interpretation* by reminding us that, because words and verbal formulations "develop from a background of sensuous experience" (p. 1), they inevitably prove limited, even reductive, when used in an attempt to describe and to convey the non-sensuously derived objects that are relevant to psychoanalytic inquiry and study. Thus, he cautions readers to be aware of the limits and inadequacy of "words and verbal formulations" (p. 1), the very things that patients and analysts are necessarily forced to resort to and rely upon: "Reason is emotion's slave and exists to rationalize emotional experience. Sometimes the function of speech is to communicate experience to another; sometimes it is to miscommunicate experience to another" (p. 1).

O and K

In Chapters 3 and 4 of *Attention and Interpretation*, Bion describes ultimate reality (O) and the domain of knowledge (K) – what can come to be known of our raw, existential Experience – and elaborates his famous injunction to try to listen to the patient without memory, desire or understanding. The latter is necessary because "established beliefs and conventions, hardened habits of thought, unless subjected to vigilance, re-establish themselves and encroach upon the freedom the psychoanalyst has won by being psycho-analysed and lead to the deterioration of his efficiency" (p. 27).

[O] stands for the absolute truth in and of any object; it is assumed that this cannot be known by any human being; it can be known about, its presence can be recognized and felt, but it cannot be known. It is possible to at one with it.

(p. 30)

O does not fall in the domain of knowledge or learning save accidentally; it can be 'become', but it cannot be 'known'. It is darkness and formlessness but it enters the domain of K when it has evolved to a point where it can be known, through knowledge gained by experience, and formulated in terms derived from sensuous experience; its existence is conjectured phenomenologically.

(p. 26)

Bion is making a plea for the exercise of the analyst's *intuition* directed towards emotions and events that are the here-and-now of the session. This is the experience that analyst and patient must try to attend to and learn from. It is the moment-to-moment truth of their encounter. If one can leave behind memory and desire, then the memories and desires that arise within the session are to be attended to as indicators of the O of the moment. They may become part of the selected fact of a given moment. But, like all extra-sessional memories and desires, they must not be clung to or they will become overvalued ideas and limit one's openness to new experience.

Language

For Bion, although discourse and language are fundamental to psychoanalysis and better than any of the available alternatives, relying upon them means trying to make the best of a bad situation. "Talking ... must be considered as potentially two different activities, one as a mode of communicating thoughts and the other as an employment of *musculature* to disencumber the personality of thoughts" (Bion 1962, p. 83).

In the latter instance, thoughts may be unconsciously felt or considered to be equivalent or analogous to concrete *things*, unwanted accretions of stimuli, because of or independent of their content. The problems that result for psychoanalysts and their patients from all of these complexities and inadequacies of language are captured in the refrain repeated by the protagonist in T.S. Eliot's (1963) poem, *Sweeney Agonistes*, about the impossibility of using words when trying to communicate deeply felt emotions to another.

Language: Communication or Evacuation

The limitations of language confound our attempts to write or talk about psychoanalysis with each other. They can become even more problematic when we offer our patients interpretations of what we feel may be happening. And yet, the need to communicate with and connect to others is fundamental to being human. Bergstein (2019) reminds us that "The urge to communicate, alongside the difficulty in communicating, seems to be the Ariadne's thread running throughout Bion's work" (Bergstein 2019, p. 98).

This observation applies to the analyst as well as the patient. 'Communicating' refers both to talking to another and trying to understand something for and often about oneself. In either case, talking or thinking may be:

- used to increase contact with reality, oneself or another;
- be used as a means of distorting one's perception of unpleasant or inconvenient facts of reality;
- avoiding the pain of ignorance and not knowing (rationalizations, falsehoods and other evasions of truth);
- used as a form of action and evacuation intended "to unburden the psyche of accretions of stimuli" (Bion 1962, pp. 28, 31) (thereby denying or destroying contact with reality or the organs of its perception).[9]

Projective Identification, Dreamwork, Container–Contained

Bion's formulation of the oeneric dimension of the mind (alpha function, waking dream thoughts and container–contained) is a theory that describes the facilitation of the growth of one's mind via the unconscious participation of another in a dyadic, transformational, intersubjective process that supports and enlarges one's capacities for containment and psychic homeostasis. While this level of participation is quite difficult to describe in words, it does indicate our need to take into consideration a dimension of the analyst's presence and actual being rather than just the words or semantic meanings of the analyst's interpretations, when thinking about the analyst's contribution to the homeostatic, psychic developmental movements mobilized in the analytic process. For Bion (1965, 1970), as for Winnicott (1965) in his famous pronouncement that there is no such thing as an infant, the extent and limits of frustration tolerance are often seen as determined by an unconscious, two-person, intersubjective process (container–contained). This is especially so in relation to the psychic development of the infant and child and in fostering the patient's psychic growth in the analytic situation.

Bion (1962) described the psyche as organized around two basic kinds of elements that he termed alpha and beta elements. The former, associated with the neurotico-normal parts of the personality, are the building blocks of thought. They can be thought with and thought about. They contribute to the *contact barrier* that separates consciousness from unconsciousness and waking life from dream life. They become psychic elements as a result of transformational work done on beta elements.

He speaks of beta elements as some kind of – or something that approximates – raw, existential Experience: unprocessed emotions and perceptions, noumena, 'things-in-themselves' (Bion 1962, 1965, 1970, 1992). These cannot be thought with or thought about, except indirectly by intuition or surmise. They may be 'felt' (e.g., they give rise to the physical aspect of the emotions), but are not yet represented psychic elements. They are associated with the psychotic part of the personality and contribute to the structure that Bion (1962) calls a *beta screen*.

In an optimal situation, beta elements are continuously being transformed by waking dreamwork (alpha function) into alpha elements, and the latter are assembled into thoughts and narratives. Throughout life, but especially in infancy and childhood, this dreamwork is continuously performed (waking and while asleep) psychically, unconsciously, autonomously and with the intersubjective assistance of primary objects. In formulating the communicative aspect of projective identification, Bion (1957, 1970) described how those disturbances (beta elements) that cannot be psychically processed, contained and metabolized autonomously are unconsciously projected into the mind of the object, where, if they are received and allowed to dwell for a long enough time, they may be 'dreamed' by the object into something that is thinkable and then re-presented to the infant/patient in some tolerable form. In this process, the infant/patient not only 'exchanges' beta elements for alpha elements, but internalizes a bit more of what will become their own, autonomous transformational capacities (alpha function). It is this intersubjectively assisted transformational system that plays a key role in Bion's formulation of therapeutic action and is central to the understanding and application of Ferro's field theory.

Beta Screen

In order to better understand the clinical implications of this formulation, it is necessary to reconsider Bion's (1962) definition of the beta screen:

> Thanks to the beta-screen the psychotic patient [– we can now add, the psychotic part of any patient –] has a capacity for *evoking emotions* in the analyst; his associations are the elements of the beta-screen intended to evoke interpretations or other responses which are less related to his need for psycho-analytic interpretation than to *his need to produce an emotional involvement*.
>
> (p. 24, italics added)

The patient's evocation of feelings in, and production of an emotional involvement with, the analyst suggest the presence of *intuition* in the patient and imply a progressive unconscious purpose and intention controlled by the non-psychotic part of the personality. The output from the beta screen has often been thought of as being only attacking, evacuative or defensive. But, looking closely at Bion's definition of beta screen and his description in the paper "On Arrogance" of his failed receptivity to the patient's projections (Bion 1957), we see that Bion was aware that the patient's aim may also be – perhaps always is! – in the service of survival: a *need to make contact by evoking feelings and an emotional involvement with the object*, because "the patient is starved of genuine therapeutic material, namely truth, and therefore ... his impulses that are directed to survival are overworked attempting to extract cure from therapeutically poor material" (Bion 1962, footnote 10.1.1., pp. 100–101).

If we view the patient's motivations from this more positive, communicative vertex, we might then see the patient's activities as unconsciously offering the analyst a course correction, unconsciously trying to recruit the analyst into having an emotional experience in order to correct for a deficient or misguided emotional involvement on the analyst's part. Or to communicate and perhaps actualize through repetition a very negative emotional experience of incomprehension or tendency to discharge tension via action (acting out) rather than thought.

In either case, what Bion is describing is not just an attack or evacuation, but a complex action that also reflects the activation of the patient's survival instinct in the face of feeling overwhelmed or deprived of emotional contact.[10] It is as if, in this way, the patient is unconsciously saying:

> I don't feel us in contact and am trying to force a connection. I can't find or use words and so can't tell you what this is I am feeling or (unsuccessfully) struggling to contain and transform, and so I am inducing something in you that perhaps you can make sense of for/with me.

This is why Bion (2005a, 2005b) often speaks about the patient as the analyst's best supervisor.

Notes

1 "Thinking starts as a personal way that the infant has for dealing with the mother's graduated failure of adaptation. Thinking is part of the mechanism by which the infant tolerates both failure of adaptation to ego-need and frustration of instinct producing tension, particularly the former" (Winnnicott 1989, p. 213).

2 Readers may notice – and perhaps will forgive – my use of a spatial metaphor here to try to convey this thought. That I have to resort to something that I know is too concrete, potentially misleading and literally 'false' – the mind is not a 'place' – is an example of the limitations of language that I am trying to speak about! For an extended discussion of this problem, see Bergstein (2019).

3 I will use the convention of using the capital E to talk about raw existential Experience, which by definition cannot be fully known, but may only 'be' or

'become,' and use the small e to refer to that part of Experience (everyday experience) that can come to be known.

4 Like Freud (see Stanicke, Zachrisson and Scarfone, 2020), Bion's epistemological reasoning rests within the Western philosophical tradition of thinkers such as Kant and Hume.

5 Laplanche (2011) describes an analogous process when he talks about the unconscious transmission, implantation and installation of an unknowable sexual desire in the creation of the infant's unconscious.

6 For further discussion, see Levine 2022 and what I have called the fundamental epistemological position.

7 See Levine, Reed and Scarfone, 2013, for a broader discussion of the unrepresented.

8 See Levine 2022 for a discussion of these problems.

9 "It is too often forgotten that the gift of speech, so centrally employed, has been elaborated as much for the purpose of concealing thought by dissimulation and lying as for the purpose of elucidating or communicating thought" (Bion 1970, p. 3).

10 Aisenstein (2017) makes an analogous assertion about somatic discharges: "Somatic outcomes are to my mind attempts – presumably last-ditch attempts – to mobilise a reparative aim in 'another', whose value as an object is at the relevant time imperceptible and uncertain" (p. 90).

References

Aisenstein, M. (2017). *An Analytic Journey.* London: Karnac.

Bergstein, A. (2019). *Bion and Meltzers' Expedition into Unmapped Mental Life.* London and New York: Routledge.

Bion, W.R. (1957). On arrogance. *International Journal of Psychoanalysis*, 39: 144–146.

Bion, W.R. (1962). *Learning from Experience.* London: Heinemann.

Bion, W.R. (1965). *Transformations.* London: Heinemann.

Bion, W.R. (1970). *Attention and Interpretation.* New York: Basic Books.

Bion, W.R. (1992). *Cogitations.* London: Karnac.

Bion, W.R. (2005a). *Tavistock Seminars.* London: Karnac.

Bion, W.R. (2005b). *Italian Seminars.* London: Karnac.

Eliot, T.S. (1963). *Collected Poems, 1909–1962.* New York: Harcourt, Brace & World.

Ferro, A. (2002). *In the Analyst's Consulting Room.* London: Routledge.

Freud, S. (1900). *The Interpretation of Dreams. Standard Edition*, Vols. 4 and 5. London: Hogarth Press.

Freud, S. (1911). *Formulations on the Two Principles of Mental Functioning. Standard Edition*, Vol. 12, pp. 213–226. London: Hogarth Press.

Laplanche, J. (2011). Starting from the fundamental anthropological situation. In: Laplanche, J. *Freud and the Sexual* (pp. 99–114). New York: International Psychoanalytic Books.

Levine, H.B. (2022). *Affect, Representation and Language. Between the Silence and the Cry.* Abingdon, UK, and New York: Routledge/IPA.

Levine, H.B., Reed, G. and Scarfone, D. (Eds.) (2013). *Unrepresented States and the Creation of Meaning.* London: Karnac/IPA.

Stanicke, E., Zachrisson, A. and Vetlesen, A.J. (2020). The epistemological stance of psychoanalysis: Revisiting the Kantian legacy. *Psychoanalytic Quarterly*, 89: 281–304.

Winnicott, D.W. (1965). The theory of the parent–infant relationship. In: Winnicott, D.W. *The Maturational Processes and the Facilitating Environment* (pp. 37–55). New York: IUP.

Winnicott, D.W. (1989). Thinking and symbol formation. In: Winnicott, D.W. *Psychoanalytic Explorations* (pp. 213–216). Ed. by C. Winnicott, R. Shepherd and M. Davis. Cambridge, MA; Harvard University Press.

Chapter 8

Memory and Desire[1]

Antònia Grimalt

Introduction

In the poem "East Coker" (1989), T.S. Eliot expresses in poetic language what Bion intends to communicate about the analyst's mental state in contact with the turbulence of the session, a state of mind that we need to develop in order to be able to keep ourselves in at-one-ness with the psychic reality (O) of the patient. Bion posits the negative capacity to train our intuition, because psychic reality has no sensory counterpart in external reality, only sensory forms of expression. Some of the latter, such as poetic language, are closer to the basis of the problem than others. Eliot expresses in his verses how preexisting knowledge, especially that based in preconceptions and repeated expectations, tends to falsify direct perception and observation and distort hope and love. He expresses, as I see it, how this 'falsified' love and hope – "structured by our habitual fears, defenses and desires" – struggle to achieve that which is already known. Then, nothing fresh, new and creative can emerge, only the repetition of old patterns.

Freud: "Free-Floating Attention"

In his "Recommendations to Physicians Practising Psycho-analysis", Freud formulates the requirement on the analyst's part to maintain "evenly distributed", or "suspended", "hovering", "circling" or "free-floating attention" and suggests that the analyst should avoid letting his observational capacity be influenced by memory. He must have full confidence in his unconscious memory and, in order not to confuse what he perceives, he must be free of expectations and desires:

> As soon as we voluntarily strain the attention with a certain intensity, we also unintentionally begin to select the material that is offered to us: we focus especially on a certain element and eliminate another, following in this selection our hopes or our tendencies. And this is precisely what we must avoid the most. If in making such a selection we allow ourselves to

DOI: 10.4324/9781032661230-9

be guided by our hopes, we run the risk of never discovering anything but what we already know and if we are guided by our tendencies, we will surely falsify the possible perception.

(Freud, 1912/1948: 326–327)

Freud argues that the principle of accepting everything with equal and balanced attention is the necessary counterpart of the rule that is imposed on the analysand by asking the latter to communicate, without criticism or selection, everything that occurs to them. Thus, he considers that, if the analyst conducts him- or herself differently, the positive results obtained by the patient's observance of "the fundamental rule" will be almost completely nullified. The analyst must avoid any conscious influence on their own retentive faculty and abandon themself entirely to their "unconscious memory". Or, rephrasing it in purely technical terms: the analyst must listen to the subject without trying to note or retain the patient's words.

We obtain the best therapeutic results in those cases in which we act as if we were not pursuing any particular goal, allowing ourselves to be surprised by each new orientation and acting freely, without prejudice … the doctor must orientate to the subject's unconscious emitter his own unconscious, as the receiving organ.

(Freud, 1912/1948: 327–328)

The metaphor of the telephone illustrates this: just as the receiver transforms back into sound waves the electrical oscillations produced by the emitted sound waves, so also the unconscious psyche of the analyst must be capable of reconstructing, with the products of the unconscious communicated to him, "this unconscious itself which has determined the occurrences of the subject". Since the psychoanalyst uses their unconscious as an instrument, they must not tolerate anything (any resistance) that would take away from their consciousness what their unconscious has discovered, for otherwise they would introduce into the analysis a new form of selection and deformation more detrimental than that which could be produced by the conscious tension of their attention.

With "the danger of never finding anything other than that which was already known", Freud makes explicit reference to the renunciation of paying attention to all conscious influences and recommends abandonment to the reception of "unconscious memory".

Avoid as far as possible all reflection and all production of conscious hypotheses; to eschew the wish to fix, especially in one's memory, anything of what he has heard, so as to apprehend in this way, with his own unconscious, the unconscious of the analysand.

(Freud, 1923/1921: 2664)

Freud speaks here of two levels:

a one referring to a very precise attitude in relation to the actual material;
b the other referring to a transformative functioning in a mental state of absence of conscious memory.

What kind of "unconscious memory" can be connected to a supposedly conscious observation capacity? With the metaphor of the telephone, he describes how the analyst has to train the receptive organ of his or her own unconscious to be able to receive and transform the "transmitting" unconscious of the patient. To my way of thinking, this has to do with the process that Bion describes with the concepts of reverie, containment and transformation, on the part of the analyst, in response to their patient's communications.

Bion (1967): "Notes on Memory and Desire"

Bion protested in private (Grotstein, 2009: 210) that everything he had written had already been said before: he simply expounded the ideas in a way that he could shed new light on them to increase their value. His aim was to revitalize concepts and metaphors that had been worn out by use and had become devitalized (Grinberg and Bea, 1991). Or, as he says in the Grid (Bion, 1971/ 1982), "to provide something akin to applying an electric shock to trivialized or widespread terms that have therefore lost their capacity to be rethought".

In 1967, Bion rescued Freud's recommendations from oblivion by discovering that the discipline of putting aside memories and desires can rescue the freshness of the analytic experience. At the same time, he unearthed "the here and now" described by Freud, a concept that Freud never used in regard to analytic technique, although his concern for the immediacy of the relationship was evident in his writings on technique.

The "only point of importance in any session is the unknown", Bion famously insisted in a short and explosive paper in 1967, "Notes on Memory and Desire". The analyst must "cultivate a watchful avoidance of memory" and avoid any desire, for results, cure, or even understanding. Psychoanalytic observation, he wrote, "is concerned neither with what has happened nor with what is going to happen but with what is happening". The only measure of 'progress' will be "the increased number and variety of moods, ideas and attitudes seen in any given session" (Bion, 1967: 17–18).

Bion published his very brief article in California in *The Psychoanalytic Forum*, where he developed Freud's approach: expectations and desires, as a potential interference in the state of openness and reception of the patient's unconscious communications, derived from memories, assumptions and preconceptions that occupy the analyst's mind. The psychoanalysts invited to comment on the article were T.M. French, J.A. Lindon, A. Gonzàlez and M. Brierley. The reactions it aroused ranged from interested reception to outright rejection. Brierley goes so far as to imply that it departs from 'correct' psychoanalytic technique. Part of this reaction was due to Bion's provocativeness and evocativeness, his tendency to use paradox, contradiction and illogic in an attempt to revitalize dead metaphors that had lost their meaning through use and abuse.

In his response to the discussions, Bion took up various points raised and broadened and specified his thought:

> Desire should not be distinguished from "memory" as I prefer that the terms should represent one phenomenon which is a suffusion of both. I have tried to express this by saying "memory" is the past tense of "desire", "anticipation" being its future tense.
>
> (Bion, 1967: 279)

> What matters to Bion is the unknown and on this he felt the psycho-analyst must focus his attention. Therefore "memory" is a dwelling on the unimportant to the exclusion of the important. Similarly, "desire" is an intrusion into the analyst's state of mind which covers up, disguises, and blinds him to the point at issue: that aspect of O that is currently presenting the unknown and unknowable though it is manifested to the two people present in its evolved character. This is the "dark spot" that must be illuminated by "blindness". Memory and desire are "illuminations" that destroy the value of the analyst's capacity for observation as a leakage of light into a camera might destroy the value of the film being exposed.
>
> (Bion, 1970/1984: 69)

The state of mind that Bion recommends to the analyst approximates what Freud described in a Letter to Lou Andreas Salomé in 1916: "I know that, in my work, I have blinded myself artificially to concentrate all the light in a dark passage". In Bion's experience, this procedure makes possible the intuition of a "present evolution" and lays the foundations for future evolutions. Part of the confusion and misunderstanding surrounding this recommendation lies in the ambiguity of the terms 'memory' and 'desire'. There is a difference between two types of phenomena that are interchangeably called 'memory':

1 a specific type of memory that Bion calls "evolution", when an idea or pictorial image emerges and floats in the mind as a whole, detached from other ideas. This experience has no sensory counterpart, although it is expressed in terms derived from the language of sensory experience. This differs from:

2 ideas that present themselves through a deliberate, conscious effort to remember, for which Bion reserves the term "memory". The former consists of an evocative or oeneric function: it appears as an occurrence and

arises from something unknown and formless as an evolution within the session. He describes it as dreamlike and stresses its quality as different from cumulative or retentive memory.

Reverie

Bion used the idea of reverie to encourage openness to the unconscious communication from the patient. At the same time, the analyst's reverie is itself a communication to the patient: the analyst who is able to maintain a state of reverie imparts something to the channels of unconscious communication themselves, just as a mother's reverie in the presence of her child is a "psychical quality ... imparted to the channels of communication, the links with the child" (Bion, 1962/1984: 36). Bion alludes to the change that takes place – a jointly experienced increase in "the number and variety of moods, ideas and attitudes" – merely by virtue of the analyst being able to maintain reverie. Throughout his work, his advice to analysts was to listen to what the patient says as if listening to a dream.

In the early 1960s, Bion characterized the analyst's capacity to sustain such listening as "alpha function", "a working tool in the analysis of disturbances of thought", which can "provide [both the analyst's and the patient's] ... psyche with the material for dream thoughts, and hence the capacity to wake up or go to sleep, to be conscious or unconscious" (Bion, 1962: 308). In doing so, Bion drew attention to the affinity between the dream and psychoanalysis itself.

Anyone who has made careful notes of what they consider to be the facts of a session must be familiar with the experience in which such notes will, on occasion, seem to be drained of all reality: they might be notes of dreams made to ensure that one will not forget them on waking. What Bion suggests is that the experience of the session relates to material akin to the dream, not in the sense that dreams might be part of the preoccupation of the session, but that the dream and the psychoanalyst's working material both share a dreamlike quality (Bion, 1970/1984: 70–71).

In his attempts to conceptualise the kind of work required for listening to the unconscious, Bion developed his mathematized 'grid'. The grid made graphic the complexity of shifting vertices in which the analyst is involved. K ('knowledge') and minus-K, L ('love'), alpha and beta were elements in an exploration of problems "fundamental to learning". His notation is an attempt to classify, think about and convey emotional experience, both the patient's and the analyst's (Bion, 1962). Bion also made use of the visual metaphor of projection in an image that seems to draw partly on theatre, with its spotlights, and partly on his experiences of war:

Instead of trying to bring a brilliant, intelligent, knowledgeable light to bear on obscure problems, I suggest we bring to bear a diminution of the "light" – a penetrating beam of darkness: a reciprocal of the searchlight.

The peculiarity of this penetrating ray is that it could be directed towards the object of our curiosity, and this object would absorb whatever light already existed, leaving the area of examination exhausted of any light that it possessed. The darkness would be so absolute that it would achieve a luminous, absolute vacuum. So that, if any object existed, however faint, it would show up very clearly. Thus, a very faint light would become visible in maximum conditions of darkness.

(Bion, 1990: 20–21)

Bion refers to memory as sensory impressions of what is supposed to have happened and desire as sensory impressions of that which has not yet happened. Observation, the cornerstone of analysis, is not about what has happened or what is going to happen, but about what is happening *now*. It thus emphasizes the centrality of the emotional experience in the session. Bion suggests that memory distorts the recording of facts because it is under the influence of unconscious forces. Desire, like memory, interferes with the intuition of the reality of the unknown. The psychoanalyst's real world deals with depression, anxiety, fear and other aspects of psychic reality. Anxiety has no form, no smell, no taste, although the emotional experience acquires form, embodied in sensations: smell, taste, sound, colors and so on. The difficulty lies in differentiating the idea, the emotion, from the sensory form that harbors it – in other words, *the map is not the territory, and the name is not the thing*. At the same time, thoughts can be treated as concrete things, without questioning their 'status' as intangibles or 'non-things'. The word 'empty' can be used to describe the state of a thought, and this does not mean that a valuable thought cannot be developed or become a profoundly destructive one.

In every psychoanalytic session there is evolution. Something evolves from the "dark and formless". This evolution may bear some resemblance to memory, but once experienced, it can never be confused with memory. It shares with dreams the quality of being totally present or suddenly absent in an inexplicable way. This evolution is what the analyst must be willing to interpret. The progress will be gauged by the increase in number and variety of moods, ideas and attitudes observed in a session.

(Bion, 1967: 280)

In his description of the communicative process and emotional climate in the session, Bion recommends thinking beyond the senses and also beyond common sense: beyond the sensory world, although we need the sensory and common sense to communicate. What we feel with our patients in the session does not come from the sensory, although the channels through which it arrives *are* sensory. The emotional experience needs a sensory or aesthetic form, detoxified of its sensory origin, which maintains the possibility of two or more vertices, allowing correlation, confrontation and binocular vision so that it can be differentiated from the 'thing-in-itself'.

> I believe that there is a psychoanalytic domain with its own reality – unquestionable, constant, subject to change only according to its own rules, even if these are not known. These realities can be intuited if there is an apparatus in proper working condition. There are a certain number of conditions necessary for its operation [...] in terms of category C, this activity depends on the presence of a personality, an intuition at work, an intuition in operation, an intuition that is a personality, a functioning intuition, a minimum degree of intuitive capacity and intuitive health [...] there are a certain number of conditions intuitive [...] the psychoanalyst should exercise his intuition in such a way that it is not damaged by the intrusion of memories, desires, or understanding.
>
> (Bion, 1992/2004: 315)

"Free floating attention" (Bion, 1992/2004: 215) can be described as the analyst's state of mind that provides the conditions in which alpha dreamwork can function to give rise to alpha elements: visual mental imagery (though not only visual; auditory 'imagery', or the abstraction of the auditory or the abstraction of a tactile or olfactory sensation) that has the specific quality which Poincaré ascribes to a selected fact. These elements must have the quality of linking the real emotional experience of the session with other fragments that, until then, "had no meaning, made no sense". The 'evolution' of the psychic will always be a brief and intense phenomenon immediately followed by the progress of the emotional flow, like the fleeting images of the dream. This state of mind intensifies one's understanding of the evolved aspects of O as 'ultimate truth/reality', a basic necessity for mental health and growth.

Following what I pointed out earlier in Freud, Bion describes two levels:

a   the receptive mental disposition observant of what is happening in the session;
b   the way in which the analyst proceeds to record, transform or interpret these events.

Bion goes further: in both situations there is a sensory register in what the analyst hears, sees, smells or feels (even in his bodily co-enesthetic posture) and receives in a state of reverie. It is a kind of sensory empathy related to the primary bond, at primitive levels of sensory register; a primary psychophysical (psychosomatic–somatopsychic) space (Bion, 1979/2000) or level of experience, where mental and physical functions present an organization at the same level;

a space where new ideas can be developed: the psychophysical texture of the lived experience lived through not yet contained psychophysical forms.

The ability to observe this register in interaction with the patient facilitates conjecture and allows intuitive discovery. It is a back-and-forth process of implicit communication that goes beyond the boundaries imposed by the intersubjective and the intrapsychic. This process of discovery requires emptying the mind of preconceived contents in order to initiate and allow a delicate, critical process of 'evolution'.

On a practical level, what it describes is a state analogous to the state of reverie of the mother with her baby. Analysts use their own "somato-psychic alpha function" in a state of reverie in order to be able to transform their patient's beta elements (basic, rudimentary proto-emotions, not mentalized) into their own personal emotions. Just as the mother "becomes a baby", the analyst "becomes a patient" in an unconscious act that transcends understanding and identification. Under these conditions, the alpha elements may become accessible to waking thought. This is what Bion calls the evolution of an alpha element (Bion, 1997), which can be used as a basis for constructing a conscious thought and become an interpretation if the analyst so chooses.

This discipline allows the analyst to be open to their own psychic objects, ephemeral, evanescent and private – insofar as they are evoked and provoked by the patient's communication and behavior (Torras de Beà, 1989). Through these objects they are able to intuit the psychic objects of the analysand. It is basically an emotional experience that, when contained by an internal alpha-parental function, gives rise to an empathic interpretation that allows the analysand to introject a creative parental partner capable of detoxifying the intolerable experience.

> I believe that if I listen to this patient, if I am prepared to hear what he has to say, if I am prepared to see what I can see if the patient comes to me, then, although the patient cannot understand what I say to him if I am using ordinary language, he may be able to understand the fact that I have not run away, I have not shut him up in a mental hospital and I am ready to arrange to see him tomorrow ... If the analyst is prepared to listen, have his eyes open, his ears open, his senses open, his intuition open, it has an effect upon the analysand who seems to grow; the session provides the mind of the patient with what, if it were a matter of physical experience, one could say was "good food".
>
> (Bion, 1990: 131)

Theoretical Pillars

In his later writings, Bion replaces his previous hypothesis about the psychotic part of the personality and goes on to speak of prenatal levels of the mind. He conjectures the existence of a thalamic terror as an explanation for certain violent human actions that do not derive from or pass through thought. His idea of a primary psychophysical space – or level of experience where mind and body share the same schema – is assimilable to Freud's "bodily ego". The conception of basic unity between psyche and soma illustrates Bion's conception of the biological, material and bodily basis of mental phenomena. By considering the patient's behavior and communication as a palimpsest of different levels of functioning, Bion argues that certain basic forms of these do not change in the adult: senso-emotional experiences or beta elements not accessible to memory and thought processes that have not been able to be transformed into alpha elements in order to be combined in dream thoughts.

People who, in their adaptive functioning, evade the crises inherent in their development, build protective structures that avoid psychic pain by splitting the emotions, which remain in a prenatal state. These emotions at the psychophysical level constitute "idées mères" as Bion calls the beta elements, when he considers them as the germ of potentialities that can evolve if they are contained and transformed. These false solutions need to find a transforming means (the receptive mind of the analyst) that attenuates the mental pain without evading it, that can give way to the psychic birth of the emotional experience. Transformation means finding meaningful words, images, expressions and/or meaning for these feelings, fantasies and/or split impressions.

Bion argues that emotional experience is ephemeral, cannot be stored, and is therefore impossible to remember; it is instantaneous and present. Only sensory experience can be remembered – that is, that which is felt and captured through one of the five senses: one can remember songs or movies or cities or perfumes that bring back evocations of moments, persons or situations, and this memory awakens an emotional experience, but this is not remembered, it is activated. Through the alpha dreamwork, the emotional experience is paired with visual images (pictograms) and transforms them into alpha elements that can be stored and remembered in the form of an ideogram that combines an emotion with a pictogram or abstraction of a sensory register. This conjunction of sensory and emotional experience occurs in different ways, evocative of past, present and future experiences that form 'the mind's eye' necessary for the imagination and insight: a cognitive emotional grammar that develops in the primary bond. The failure of this grammar as an intuitive 'matrix of the self' manifests itself in the form of emotional disconnection and isolation (Grimalt, 2004).

To summarize:

a   *Emotional* experience is unrepeatable and unstorable. One can 'remember' an experience that is sufficiently close to the emotional experience we expect to find associated with a specific situation, but it will never be the same as that experience: the new experience is completely new; what remains is the evocative remnant of the associated sensory experience.

b   In contrast, the sensory experience *can* be stored and thought. It has a highly evocative component and tends to be saturated with meaning.

c   (c) Alpha dreamwork is the process by which emotional experience, which cannot be processed or stored, is transformed into thinkable sensory experience. It is probably because of this surplus of emotional experience that it is impossible to transmit the dreamed dream. It is in this surplus that Bion says that the emotional experience dwells: that which evaporates when transforming the emotional experience into sensorial experience.

As we know, with his approach to alpha dreamwork, Bion offers a different version of Freud's concept of dreamwork:

> The psychoanalytic use of the dream as a method by which the unconscious becomes conscious, constitutes a reversed use of that which in reality constitutes the mechanism used in transformation of conscious material into material suitable for storage in the unconscious. In other words, the dreamwork constitutes but a small part of the dreaming proper, which is a continuous process that belongs to waking life and acts during waking hours, but which is not usually observed except in the psychotic patient.
>
> (Bion, 1992/2004)

In this context, the nocturnal sleep is part of a process of digestion of an indigestible emotional experience that is linked to a daytime remnant to be evoked in images. Not only does the dream reveal the unconscious, but all emotional experiences need to be dreamed in order to be transformed into something knowable. The transformations, inherent in mental functioning, must be learned (from experience) by the analyst who trains their mind to perform this process in real time. Bion calls the state of mind suitable for dreaming the patient's content *faith*, and notes that it is associated with the renunciation of memory, desire and understanding. Memory limits the plasticity of the mental container. The hasty understanding of something makes it difficult to tolerate that the phenomenon may have no meaning. And desires, like voracious containers, search in the analytic medium for certain predetermined contents in order to rationalize and confirm a theory.

The common sense of clinical experience indicates that the more attentive we are to the appearance of certain content, the more prone we are to produce it. The analytical sense that allows us to get around the obstacles that our desire produces requires intuition, which rummages in the depths of the material in search of the facts, the truth that lies hidden there. Bion's description alerts us to the danger of the patient becoming a theoretical fiction of the analyst or the analyst shielding him- or herself behind a defensive theoretical barrier to avoid the anxiety of contact with the patient:

> The objection to memory can be sustained because all memory is a special case of (keeping) possessing a theory that is known (or suspected) to

be false to avoid the psychological disorder that always accompanies mental development.

(Bion, 1970/1984: 35)

In Chapter 4 of *Attention and Interpretation* Bion (1970/1984) makes his technical reasons explicit. He observes that, if the analyst remembers some specific type of data about the patient, they reduce their perspective because they cannot be free to make use of their intuition through free-floating attention. Recollection can be seen as an anticipatory suppression of surprise in the face of the unknown. His emphasis on disciplining desire proceeds from the observation that subjection to the pleasure principle prevents observing the patient as he or she is and the level at which he or she functions, which may not be what we would like it to be. The exercise of letting go of understanding is also related to both. What is meant by understanding is the rush to take something for granted, thereby restricting the possibility of observing, respecting and taking time to listen to the patient's opinions, theories and explanations. The analytic situation requires intuition and apprehension, rather than hasty understanding. All three are the product of denial of the unknown, anxiety and haste (Sandler, 2005).

If the analyst uses intuition to follow the evolution of the patient's psychic state in the session, the analyst's interpretations should gain in strength and conviction – both for themself and for the patient – because they derive from emotional experience with a unique individual, and not from imperfect generalized theories. Similarly, Freud speaks of artificial blinding. As a method of arriving at this artificial blindness, Bion points out the importance of avoiding memory and desire. To continue and extend the process, Bion includes the avoidance of understanding and sensory perception among the properties to be avoided.

The suspension of memory, desire, comprehension and sensory impressions may seem impossible without a complete negation of reality, but the psychoanalyst is looking for something different from what is usually known as reality: an attitude directed toward making contact with psychic reality – that is, the evolved characteristics of O. This procedure is valid in psychoanalysis and other sciences; likewise, F (faith) is an essential component of the scientific procedure, however rigorous it may be (Bion, 1970/1984: 45).

Intuition, as a preconscious, non-discursive thought process, is the basis of creativity. As I see it, Bion conceives it as a way of integrating an archaic way of co-enesthetic thinking, which implies a kind of global instinctive resource to deal with various undifferentiated phenomena such as forms, shadows, multidimensionality, independent of the boundaries between sensory modalities. It can become difficult to translate intuitive experiences into verbal forms but, when successful, subtle penumbras of meaning in linguistic content and prosody are conveyed. However, these observations require rational exploration to be confirmed. Following Kant, Bion considers that "intuition without concept is blind; concept without intuition is empty".

Intuition as an essential instrument of the psychoanalyst is also used in the service of creating a space and form adequate to the interpretation. I believe that Bion gives shape to a kind of internal ethics regarding the way of the creative, versus defensive or destructive way of relating to thoughts. In a beautiful and dense cogitation (Bion, 1992/2004: 125), he posits compassion and truth as human senses (signifying psychic faculties analogous to sensory perception) exercised, expected and sought in interaction with the other. He differentiates between interpretation, as propaganda, and the interpretation arising from a transformative process of the emotional experience with the patient and comments that one should not interpret something that one does not feel.

There are silences that are nothing, they are 0, zero. But sometimes the silence becomes something fruitful and becomes 101 – the previous sounds and the ones that follow make it a valuable communication, just like the silences and pauses in music, and gaps and spaces in sculpture.

Gooch (2001) vividly describes the essence of Bion's ideas on theory and practice of the psychoanalytic technique, based on his personal experience; he considers that, when analysts makes accurate and heartfelt verbal interpretations, using their own psychic objects, in words – like the lyric of a song – they integrate aspects of music and dance in an authentic way. It is the music and dance of interpretation that makes possible the transformation of the childlike aspects of the patient (Caper, 2020).

The negative capability to exist amid uncertainties, mysteries, doubts without becoming obsessed with reaching for facts and reasons is what the analyst needs in order to be in unity with himself and with the patient's emotional experience. Bion associates it with a language of unsaturated quality, which promotes evolving transformations toward the development of the expression of emotional experience. This language of artistic and scientific variations has the capacity to cross caesuras of time and space. Bion contrasts this 'language of achievement' with the language of substitution, used as a substitute for thought and not as a prelude to the communication of thought. The imaginative capacity derives from the link between analytical intuition and the language of realization, developed (Bion, 1970/1984) from the act of faith (F) or scientific state of mind of analysis – that is, without desire, without memory and without the need to understand.

So, Bion proposes to develop "negative capability" to tolerate the sensation of fragmentation and to contain it until something clearer emerges (from faith in evolution). But, with this disposition, one becomes more vulnerable to the projective identifications of the patient. This is why the analyst tends to defensively seek a logical knowledge of "facts and reasons" that make observation difficult. When analysts finds themselves in a state of reverie, keeping at bay (as much as possible) memory and desire, it means that they are more receptive to their own observations of the patient and to the emergence of 'evolutions' of their own alpha elements at the conscious level (and other unconscious mental activity, including complex thoughts).

When the analyst 'empties' or 'unsaturates' their mind of that which is 'known', a delicate and critical process of emotional growth begins. The process can be feared as catastrophic: the previous meaning has to be deconstructed before a new meaning is constructed.

The conscious, active effort to abstain from memory and desire leads the analyst to feel helpless on many levels and in many dimensions, because they are embracing experience without protective theoretical umbrellas. In the bidirectional oscillation between the schizoparanoid and depressive positions, the insight does not take place simply by the progressive construction of manageable experience. The analytic task involves coping with episodes of meaninglessness ("beta elements"), alternating with the turbulent process of containment, emotional thinking and productive evocation of alpha elements that allow for the transformation of experience.

Both Bion and Freud speak of the quality of the analyst's attention – the extent to which their theoretical preconceptions impose themselves on their mind, on their perspectives on the patient, and how the account of the patient's history can condition their listening. Freud considered neurosis a disease of memories. For Bion, the essence of the psychoanalytic process is transformative and catalytic, rather than decodifying; it is based not on reviewing past experiences but on "having present experiences". Thinking does not consist in organizing feelings in retrospect but in accessing current feelings, which are 'present' and are 'transformed' into symbols through the alpha function, a complex multilevel process that goes from sensation to the first sketches of thought.

Bion's approach is closely linked to that of transformation in hallucinosis which, in its broadest sense, has to do with predetermination: the patient sustains their independence from everything other than their own creations and creates a perfect and superior world. Under such circumstances, any frustration is experienced as a hostile or envious attack. I think that the discipline Bion recommends is aimed at preventing the analyst, at a certain level, from also being able to make transformations in hallucinosis by seeing in the patient that which they project onto the patient according to their theories, emotional needs and personal narratives. If the analyst abandons the observation of unknown facts that are revealed in the session, what is left is an overreliance on memories, or theories. In the same way that Freud speaks of "blind spots", I think we could also speak of "points in hallucinosis". I agree with Virginia Ungar (2009) that analysts should take into account not only what they cannot see, but also that which is attributed to perception when, in fact, its origin lies in the psyche. This is an important point: the projective aspect of perception (at the mental level) can become the basis for the concept of transformation in hallucinosis.

Repercussions and Developments in Technique

It is said that the richness of an idea lies in its capacity to generate new ideas. I believe that, with the development of the communicative aspect of Klein's projective identification through the relation container–content (♂♀), Bion opens up important perspectives. The discipline he recommends is at the service of a kind of 'presence' that maximizes the capacities for observation of experience in the 'here and now of the session'. Hence, he considers that memory and desire vividly and pervasively obstruct emotional experience when what we are dealing with is a kind of 'presence', a kind of careful perception–containment–transformation that is less tinged by our own narcissistic tendencies and defensive identification with our theories.

> In a session I am interested in what I do not know. The session is the only time where I can have contact with what I don't know; at any other time, I can only have contact with, or think about, phenomena that I believe – rightly or wrongly – to be true – that I have already observed or have observed only partially. It is an opportunity that cannot be missed, because it can never be repeated. It therefore deserves a description as precise as possible to delineate the emotional experience that I consider of the utmost importance. It is the right experience for the observation of a series of apparently unrelated facts that the analyst considers to be related to each other and to him in a meaningful way. At first glance it seems obvious that this emotional experience resembles the schizoparanoid position. But just because it resembles it does not mean that it is the same because it would avoid the possibility of synthesis, which is essential to the analyst's work.
>
> (Bion, 1992/2004: 215)

In regard to the analyst's preferred listening stance, Bion writes:

> I have coined the term "patience". My intention is that it retains its association with suffering and tolerance of frustration. Patience should be retained without "an exacerbated eagerness to come to fact and reason" until a pattern evolves. This state is similar to what Melanie Klein calls the depressive position. For this state I use the term "security" ... I consider the experience of oscillating between "patience" and "security" is an indication that valuable work is being done.
>
> (Bion, 1970/1984)

The communication of the transformed experience of the session, through interpretation, is always limited by something that remains beyond the sensory, the O space of the multi-dimensional psychic reality, the surplus of emotional experience that evaporates in the transformation. Neuman (2010) points out the price that must be paid for substituting the pre-symbolic lexicon of the highly dimensional unconscious, linked to emotion, with a symbolic representation of low dimensionality. This price is reification: the objectification of the lived experience and the draining of its vitality and complexity.

The patient may feel the analyst's desire as something that obstructs their authentic evolution. It could be said that the analyst's desire determines a 'preconceived form', a style of care for the patient, when the patient, in and of themselves, often seeks to adapt to what the analyst supposedly expects of them. The less the analyst identifies themself with desires or expectations, the better they will be able to analyze the expectations or desires projected by the patient. The greater the fluency to open up to the unknown and to tolerate a state of uncertainty, the more the analytic partner's mental space of the analytic couple and the possible transformations of the patient and analyst will be greatly expanded.

One could say, as in Eliot's poem, that being without memory and desire is like recognizing the space between two thoughts (or between two scenes, in the darkness of the change of scenery) while remaining in this 'interval' in a 'moment of presence' from which evolves the capacity to choose or decide. Or what Bion calls the (counter-trans)ference, pointing out the relationship between objects rather than some qualities of the objects themselves. I think this process is so powerful and, at the same time, so subtle that the essential work of the analyst consists first of all in focusing attention on what is happening in the session or on the nature of what is being experienced – how they feel emotionally pushed or drawn to experience or behave in a certain way.

Conclusion

Through experiencing Freud's "free-floating attention", Bion considers that the analytic relationship is revitalized when memories of previous sessions and theoretical preconceptions are set aside. His complex and difficult discipline involves greater solitude, with no theoretical handholds, to be receptive to evolution and discovery. His preferred listening stance deconstructs meaning through the systematic use of the dynamic reversible perspective. It destabilizes the opposition of concepts to provoke a creative tension that generates new thoughts.

Thus, Bion takes theory and technique into the realm of indeterminism, complexity and uncertainty and subordinates the drive orientation to an ontological (emotional) epistemology.

By means of the technique of surprising the reader, Bion achieves the transition to an aesthetic paradigm-centered emotional experience. In consonance with the theory of relativity and the principle of uncertainty, he proposes a new psychoanalytic paradigm that implies the idea of absolute truth about an infinite reality, absolute truth about an uncertain (chaotic) and noncognizable infinite reality that intersects with emotional boundaries. This raises the contrast between the immensity of mental space and the three-dimensional spatial-temporal order introduced by the activation of the thinking functions. It configures the catastrophic as a conflict between the intensity of the emotion and the restrictive character of the representation –

representation that can lead to paralysis or inhibition of mental resources, or end in catastrophe when the excessive emotion cannot be contained.

Free association and free-floating attention are not free at all; they are simply determined by unconscious drives and motives rather than by conscious intentions. At no point does Bion say that being without memory or desire can't be achieved at all, but rather that it is a discipline to try to do so. He simply tries to get to the basis of lived experience without opacities that obstruct intuition, so basic to our mental work when we use the psycho-analytic function of the personality.

Bion put much emphasis on intuition, relating it to the "passionate" link between two minds or to psychic reality itself. In reality, the motive underlying the discipline of containing memories, desires and 'understanding' is to contribute to the intuitive contact with the evolving psychic reality. Used in a fetishistic way, however, one might speak of non-memory and non-desire as concrete possessions and use the negation that comes with the idea of possession of a concept or attitude as if it were a 'thing' and thus destroy its meaning.

In "Making the Best of a Bad Job" (1979/2000), Bion posits three vital principles: Feeling, thinking (in the sense of alpha function) and Thinking (capitalized, in the sense of conscious function). I see this as a qualitative way of describing the capacity to feel, tolerate and contain the emotional storm of mental contact with the patient; to make the best of feelings and thoughts without barriers; to tolerate the dangerous emotional experience of the encounter with the pre- and postnatal parts of the personality by transforming them through alpha dreamwork. This implies an analysis which does not exclude the intuition of the more primitive aspects of the mind, tolerating non-comprehension and uncertainty in the hopeful search for new ideas and trying to communicate them in a creative way.

Note

1   A previous version of this paper was published in the review *Temas de Psicoanalisis*: "Memoria y deseo" en el pensamiento de Bion. Vigencia teórica y técnica. Dossier 1 (2011).

References

Bion, W.R. (1962/1984). *Learning from Experience*. London: Karnac.
Bion, W.R. (1962). The Psycho-Analytic Study of Thinking. *International Journal of Psycho-Analysis*, 43: 306–310.
Bion, W.R. (1967). Notes on Memory and Desire. *The Psychoanalytic Forum*, 2: 271–280.
Bion, W.R. (1970/1984). *Attention and Interpretation*. London: Karnac.
Bion, W.R. (1971/1982). *La Tabla y la Cesura*. Buenos Aires: Gedisa.
Bion, W.R. (1979/2000). Making the Best of a Bad Job. In *Clinical Seminars and Other Works*. London: Karnac.

Bion, W.R. (1990/2014). *A Memoir of the Future*. In The Complete Works of W.R. Bion. London: Routledge.

Bion, W.R. (1997). *Taming Wild Thoughts*. Ed. by F. Bion. London. Karnac.

Bion, W.R. (1992/2004). *Cogitations*. Ed. by F. Bion. London. Karnac.

Caper, R. (2020). *Bion and Thoughts Too Deep For Words*. London and New York: Routledge.

Eliot, T.S. (1989). *Four Quartets* (trans. J.E. Pacheco). Mexico: Fondo de cultura económica.

Freud, S. (1912/1948). *Advice to the Physician in Psychoanalytic Treatment*. In Collected Works, Vol. II. Madrid: Biblioteca nueva.

Freud, S. (1923/1981). Psychoanalysis [two encyclopedia articles]. In Collected Works, Vol. III. Madrid. Biblioteca nueva.

Gooch, J.S. (2001, July). Bion's Perspectives on Psychoanalytic Technique. Panel presented in the IPA Congress in Nice.

Grimalt, A. (2004). Falsos contenidors de l'experiència emocional. *Revista Catalana de psicoanàlisi*, XXI(1–2): 139–154.

Grinberg, L. and Bea, J. (1991). *Seminario sobre el pensamiento de Bion*. Barcelona: Institut de psicoanàlisi de Barcelona.

Grotstein, J. (2009). *But at the Same Time and on Another Level: Psychoanalytic Theory and Technique in the Kleinian/Bionian Mode*. Vol. 1. London and New York: Routledge.

Neuman, Y. (2010). Penultimate Interpretation. *International Journal of Psycho-Analysis*, 91: 1043–1054.

Sandler, P.C. (2005). *The Language of Bion. A dictionary of concepts*. London: Karnac.

Torras de Beà, E. (1989). Projective Identification and Differentiation. *International Journal of Psycho-Analysis*, 70: 265–274.

Ungar, V. (2009). Discusión del panel sobre observación de bebés presentado en Boston. At Conference on Bion, Crecimiento y turbulencia emocional.

Chapter 9

Caesura

A Close Reading Seminar of Bion's Text

Avner Bergstein

I would like to read some parts of Bion's text with you and offer some of my thoughts about it. This is a paper we could talk about for years, but, since we only have a short time, we can just read a number of excerpts. Moreover, this paper seems to contain almost all of Bion's ideas throughout the years. They are all condensed in this one short paper. Nevertheless, I would like to draw attention to a number of points which I see as the most significant ones.

This paper was published in 1977. However, Bion presented this text in a number of conferences in different versions (cf. Aguayo, 2013). Moreover, Bion discussed these ideas and the notion of caesura in the 1970s, from several different vertices, in the many seminars he held, in Rome, Brazil, the Tavistock, and many other places. When we read this paper itself, many parts may be difficult to comprehend, but, if we read what he writes throughout these years from different perspectives, we begin to have a more integrated and comprehensive view of what he is trying to convey and, thus, get closer to the essence of his thinking.

In a similar vein, the paper itself begins with ten citations from different perspectives, or vertices, of which we will read just one. These citations illustrate a similar notion from different disciplines, namely psychoanalysis, Jewish mysticism, Catholic mysticism, even a book on microeconomics, all trying to depict the same idea. The most important is Freud's statement from *Inhibitions, Symptoms and Anxiety*, which you are probably all familiar with: "There is much more continuity between intra-uterine life and earliest infancy than the impressive caesura of the act of birth allows us to believe" (Freud, 1926, p. 138).

Caesura is a word Freud borrows from literature – prosody and poetry. The word denotes a break after which there is continuity, much like in a poem where you have a verse that ends in mid-sentence and continues in the following line. There's a break, but there is a continuity.

Bion writes:

> The foregoing quotations were made from the vertex of different disciplines, at different times and in different languages. They delineate the universe of discourse within which this paper is confined.

DOI: 10.4324/9781032661230-10

Psycho-analysis is concerned with the domain of ideas; included are thoughts and feelings of all kinds. Although it could be described as a limited domain, a limited human activity, its scope nevertheless is vast when one considers all thoughts, feelings and ideas which are presented to us in the course of our work. In the physical sciences the human being is dealing with a physical material: psychoanalysts are concerned with characters, personalities, thoughts, ideas and feelings. But whatever the discipline there is a primitive, fundamental, unalterable and basic line – the truth. "What is truth?" said jesting Pilate, according to Francis Bacon, and would not wait for an answer. We probably cannot wait for an answer, because we have not the time. Nevertheless, that is what we are concerned with – inescapably and unavoidably – even if we have no idea what is true and what is not. Since we are dealing with human characters we are also concerned with lies, deceptions, evasions, fictions, phantasies, visions, hallucinations – indeed, the list can be lengthened almost indefinitely.

(Bion, 1977/1989, pp. 41–42)

In this introductory passage, Bion seems to tell us almost everything he will go on to say in this paper. First, as mentioned before, he says something about these quotations taken from different vertices, and already, by that, he seems to be responding to the question "what is truth?"

Bion does not talk about *the* truth, but about *a sense* of truth. It seems he brings us all these quotations at the beginning not only to show the affinity between different disciplines, but to stress the notion that, when an idea, or an experience, is repeated over and over in several disciplines, the correlation between them affords a sense of truth. This is something Bion already writes about in 1962 at the end of his paper "A Theory of Thinking":

a sense of truth is experienced if the view of an object which is hated can be conjoined to a view of the same object when it is loved and the conjunction confirms that the object experienced by different emotions is the same object. A correlation is established.

A similar correlation, made possible by bringing conscious and unconscious to bear on the phenomena of the consulting room, gives to psycho-analytic objects a reality that is quite unmistakable even though their very existence has been disputed.

(Bion, 1962/1967, p. 119)

This point runs throughout "Caesura", suggesting that achieving a sense of truth necessitates the observation of the psychoanalytic object from different vertices, the important point being *movement*. The *invariance* becomes apparent through this perpetual movement between different vertices, and when these experiences are repeated over time. For example, if I watch a movie, and there's something there which echoes something I have read in a psychoanalytic paper, I might have a powerful emotional experience, an immediate feeling of its truthfulness. This is reminiscent of Freud's notion of a sense of "conviction" that something is true, which one achieves in analysis.

Moreover, in this paragraph, Bion seems to be talking about the caesura between material and psychic aspects of reality. Although we are emphasizing *psychic* reality, it is only one more view of reality. We must remember that Bion always talks about reality being sensuous *and* psychic, in complex dialectic interplay. He is not talking about one opposed to the other, but about different facets of the same ultimate reality. At each moment, we observe the patient from a different perspective. We realize that the patient is not exactly the same patient they were the previous session, and yet, it is, nevertheless, the same patient. Transformation *and* invariance. Observing the patient from different vertices, through their perpetual transformations, allows us to approach, over time, the invariance of the encounter with that specific patient, an invariance that feels truthful.

Let us read on:

> In our relationships with analysands time is limited and choice inescapable. Which, of all the right interpretations, are we to choose to formulate? The analyst's freedom, though great, can be seen to be limited, at any rate on one boundary, by the need to be truthful, to give an interpretation which is a true one. If the analysand is sincere in his wish for treatment he likewise is limited; his free association should be as near to what he considers to be the truth as he can get. The course of the discussion itself between analyst and analysand may make it more possible to assess the degree of truth or falsity in any particular idea which is under scrutiny.
>
> (Bion, 1977/1989, p. 42)

Bion seems to be highlighting the fact that reality is infinite. There are infinite vertices from which to observe the ultimate reality of the session. How are we to know which vertex to observe from?

Bion is also acknowledging *the need* for caesuras, the need to make choices. Which interpretation are we to give? Can any growth take place *without* caesuras? Without splitting? Without repression? But how do we know where to make the caesura. This he tries to elaborate here, again stressing the *movement* between different caesuras.

So, the first vertex from which Bion seems to be talking is that of *movement and the need to observe from different vertices*.

He now moves to another vertex and writes:

> The embryologist speaks about 'optic pits' and 'auditory pits'. Is it possible for us, as psychoanalysts, to think that there may still be vestiges in

the human being which would suggest a survival in the human mind, analogous to that in the human body, of evidence in the field of optics that once there were optic pits, or in the field of hearing that once there were auditory pits? Is there any part of the human mind which still betrays signs of an 'embryological' intuition, either visual or auditory?

This may seem to be an academic and unimportant matter – unless we think that there may be some truth in the statement made by Freud that there is some connection between post-natal thought and emotional life, and prenatal life. To exaggerate the question for the sake of simplicity: are we to consider that the foetus thinks, or feels, or sees, or hears? If so, how primitive can these thoughts, or feelings, or ideas be?

(Bion, 1977/1989, p. 42)

Often, this part of his writings is thought about as if Bion is saying that mental life begins in utero, before birth. That may be true. However, I do not think that is the main point. I don't think he is presenting a developmental theory of the personality, but rather, a theory of psychoanalytical *observation*. We must remember that the caesura between pre- and postnatal life is for Bion but *a model*, a metaphor. It seems to me he is trying to say that we find all kinds of vestiges in the realms of the body, that is, remains of some bodily organ that might have existed in utero, although, over time, it might have lost its necessity or function and ultimately disappeared. Yet still, *something*, perhaps sensuously invisible, has nevertheless remained that betrays its existence. Is it possible, he asks, that the same happens in the mind? Could there be something in the mind which also dates back to times, or levels of existence, that are very far away and invisible to our senses and yet are still psychically present in some form? To my mind, this is not said in order to discuss life in utero, or to understand some phenomenon we later see in adult life. Perhaps that too. However, Bion is using the caesura of birth as a metaphor for all that is concealed from our observation. He is actually talking about how, in analysis, we may be engrossed in the sensuously visible; there are so many things that are precluding us from seeing *beyond*. First and foremost is verbal communication itself, that is, the words themselves, which are so impressive that we get caught up in them.

In fact, in the quotation "there is much more continuity between intra-uterine life and earliest infancy than the impressive caesura of the act of birth allows us to believe", the most important word for Bion is "impressive". At times, something might be so impressive that it blinds us to seeing some other thing in the ultimate reality of the session. A patient may arrive at their session and tell of something terrible that happened on the way, or yesterday, in external life, outside the room. The story may be so impressive that we are deluded into thinking that the patient is talking about that. However, as Bion writes, this may be what the patient is *saying*. But, "what [is] the patient talking *about*?" (Bion, 1965a/1984, p. 17). No doubt they *are* talking about that, but not *only* about that. Can we extend our universe of discourse beyond the finite, restricted world within our sight and move towards an *infinite* universe of discourse? Are we going to be able to see beyond these impressive caesuras, these stories from the past and those we wish for in the future? Beyond the memories and desires, our own and the patient's? Beyond the caesuras of past and future, in order to see the emotional turbulence present before our eyes, and yet invisible to us on account of the impressive narrative stories we are confronted by?

Bion is trying to say that the so-called psychotic part of the personality, whose capacity for thinking is deficient, may often be disguised as a non-psychotic part, using apparently symbolic language to describe something which may in fact be unrepresentable and ineffable. We listen to the words the patient speaks in a most articulate way, but they may also deafen us to the emotional turbulence in the room, in the present, between the patient and ourselves. The emotional turbulence may be so disturbing, or painful, that it might be easier to grasp onto something very impressive the patient is telling, and so an impenetrable caesura is created beyond which we cannot see. And, in that sense, it becomes, in fact, a rupture, not a caesura.

The concept of caesura tries to address the barriers that might be erected in the room, which are so impressive that we are unable to see beyond them. The caesura of birth is thus only a metaphor for that.

Bion writes in *Transformations*:

> Superficially, an analytic session may appear boring, or featureless, alarming, or devoid of interest, good or bad. The analyst, seeing beyond the superficial, is aware that he is in the presence of intense emotion; there should be no occasion on which this is not apparent to him.
>
> The intense experience is ineffable but once known cannot be mistaken ...
>
> One such group of superficialities pertains to the circumstances in which analysis is conducted. These are usually physically comfortable and bear the stamp of unadventurous civilized existence. They therefore conspire against awareness that analysand and analyst are engaged on a venture which is as hazardous as activities in which the perils are more obvious and dramatic. In what the danger consists will depend on circumstances, but danger and awareness of danger are features of the situation with which the analyst should be in contact. The approach to it, to be effective, is 'binocular'; the analyst must be aware, while attending to the patient's material, of the dangers of his association with that particular patient: he should also be able to see what the danger is that the patient is inviting him by his presence to share.
>
> (Bion, 1965/1984, pp. 74–75)

Here again, Bion writes of the delusion created by the analytic session, by the comfortable couch, temperature, and so on, where this apparently innocent conversation between two people, too often on quiet waters, in fact hides the intense emotional turbulence lurking beyond the caesura of the superficial calm that we are observing.

So, that is the second vertex I would like to highlight – *the caesura of birth as a metaphor for all that is concealed from our view.*

Bion goes on to say:

> Events sometimes take place in the consulting room, where there are present only myself and a grown man or woman, which suggest feelings that I could describe as envy, love, hate, sex, but which seem to have an intense and unformed character.
>
> (Bion, 1977/1989, pp. 42–43)

Bion seems to be telling us something about the encounter with what he denotes as the psychotic part of the personality; but this term is very misleading, because we tend to hear the word 'psychotic' from the vertex of psychopathology. Bion does not seem to talk about it in that sense alone, but rather about those emotional realms of experience which cannot be verbally articulated and which are peculiar to the psychotic personality on account of their deficient capacity for verbal thought. Bion seems to be saying that, when we are in the room with a patient, we are confronted by an emotional experience that is often formless and very unformulated. There is *something* in the room which we can feel at the tip of our fingers. We may feel there is something very intense and yet we cannot find words for it. We may be confronted by the unrepressed unconscious, something which is unconscious but as yet unmentalized, undifferentiated and unknown. Bion reminds us that it is easy to fall back on familiar, saturated words. For example, when confronted with this turmoil in the analytic session, which we find completely incomprehensible, we are lost and might then resort to saying "the patient is attacking my mind" or "the patient attacks the linking". These words delude us into thinking we understand what is going on, when in fact we have no idea. We find ourselves facing something which is completely unknown, or unknowable, to us. This is an example of a caesura which we need to find a way to transcend. Bion stresses how hard it is for us to penetrate what "we all know". He suggests there might be something as yet unknown that has not emerged from the turbulence. He further tries to describe those feelings we are immersed in and yet cannot find any words for, suggesting we need to find new, unsaturated terms which will compel us to pause and think again.

He goes on to say:

> It is convenient to fall back on physiology and anatomy to borrow ideas in order to express my feelings about some of these events; to think of some of the feelings which the patient is expressing as being subthalamic, or sympathetic, or para-sympathetic.
>
> (Bion, 1977/1989, p. 43)

Bion seems to be trying to find a language for thinking about the ineffable. He reaches out to anatomy to borrow some words which, although inadequate, and albeit being somewhat strange or even bizarre, might nevertheless convey a sense of *something* that might correspond to what he is trying to describe. We should therefore not try to understand these words in their semantic, lexical meaning. Rather, these words serve to evoke an emotional experience which Bion tries to help us get in touch with. In his *Clinical Seminars* he writes:

> I wish it were possible to discuss these matters without having to invent a language as if it were scientifically accurate. But it is the best we can do until such time as it becomes possible to use it scientifically. It is useful to consider "subthalamic" fear, meaning by that any of these emotions which have not risen to the point where they could be called "conceptualized", or conscious, or verbalizable.
>
> (Bion, 1976a/1994, p. 273)

Bion implores that we will not be deluded by these words as if they were describing some scientific-neurological phenomenon, but rather use these words as what might be called "scientific-fictions" (Bion, 1976b/1994, p. 308) in order to talk about that which may be unverbalizable.

This may be one more reason for bringing those quotations at the beginning of the paper, as if saying that the discussion of ineffable emotional or theoretical experience necessitates borrowing words from other disciplines which might help convey what one is trying to express. As Bion writes,

> certain problems may be handled by mathematics, others by economics, others by religion. It should be possible to transfer a problem that fails to yield to the discipline to which it appears to belong to a discipline that *can* handle it.
>
> (1970/1984, p. 91)

To that end, Bion borrows concepts from Kant, from Plato, from St John of the Cross, from mathematicians, from neurology and so on. Regrettably, we find many papers arguing that Bion misinterpreted Kant, or Plato, or mysticism, and so on. But that is of no importance. Bion claims he does not purport to teach us any of those disciplines or philosophical ideas. He is using words which, for him, echo something he wants to express. As he said, if he finds a phrase that is helpful to him, or that someone has managed to formulate well something which he can't formulate any better, he would like to take it and use it *for his own purposes*. Moreover, by borrowing these words, he seems to illustrate the power of concepts to evoke an experience which does not necessarily coincide with the semantic, lexical meaning.

He continues:

> There are occasions when the patient mentions some anxiety, fear, or a symptom (like blushing) briefly and unobtrusively, yet in a way which suggests that something is being mentioned in disguised and feeble terms because it is the best that the patient can do to give effect to feelings which are feared for their intensity, magnitude and obtrusiveness compared with those feelings which most people are used to regard as normal.
>
> (Bion, 1977/1989, p. 43)

We might observe a blush, or perhaps notice an *apparently* unrelated nuance. Could this be the only way available for a patient to express some experience for which they have no words? Bion again cautions us from rushing in with a precocious, seemingly obvious interpretation – for example, that the patient is blushing because they are embarrassed. Perhaps, Bion speculatively conjectures, blushing is the reciprocal of turning pale with dread or anxiety. Could we play with our observations without rushing to a preconceived explanation? Could we attend to these faint experiences, which may seem insignificant, or inexplicable, but which may nevertheless be the patient's unconscious way of expressing an experience which has never been mentalized and, hence, has not been repressed? Bion thus refers to an "inaccessible" state of mind, experiences not registered mentally, which nonetheless still betray an inchoate mental life, so concealed, so encapsulated, unverbalizable, that the person themself cannot find an articulate way of expressing it.

He goes on to say: "These things, so faintly expressed, may in truth be very powerful ... and which can hardly be said to belong to what we call 'thought'" (Bion, 1977/1989, p. 43).

Bion refers to these 'things', which he denotes as β-elements, as something which does not really fall into the category of thought. And yet, he wonders whether we could extend our ordinary meaning and understanding of the term 'thought' and think of these β-elements as elements of the personality which are just not perceptible to us in the ordinary way and yet evoke a very strong experience in the analyst. We are then immersed in a hazy, 'gaseous' experience, sensuously invisible and yet powerful enough to produce an emotional involvement which cannot be explained away as 'countertransference'. We are used to thinking about 'thoughts' as something mental, but could there be thoughts which are expressed in a different way, *apparently* incomprehensible? Bion always reiterates the need to be cautious not to impose our rational, awake logic so as to assume we understand something which is of a different logic, the logic of the unconscious, or perhaps that of intrauterine life.

Bion says:

> If you apply pressure to your eyeball you can see, in response to the physical pressure, what appears to be something which could only be a

response of the optic apparatus. If that is so then maybe the optic pits respond to pressure even before the dramatic caesura of birth itself. From the point of view of the analyst the fact that the analysand is a grown man or woman can be so obtrusive, the evidence of the eyes so obtrusive, that it blinds him to feelings which are not so clearly presented to the optic apparatus.

(Bion, 1977/1989, p. 43)

We are so accustomed to thinking that we can rely on our sense of sight for deciphering reality. Could we think about the embryo's experience when, for example, the fluctuations in the amniotic fluid apply pressure on the eyeballs. This pressure generates shadows, colors, sights, just like when we shut our eyes and apply pressure onto our eyelids, subsequently 'seeing' all kinds of 'sights'. If so, what does the fetus do with it? Where are these experiences registered in the absence of a capacity to mentalize or register? Or, in Bion's words, "the poet hadn't turned up; so the recording tape was a blank!" (Bion, 1975/1991, p. 120). We see a grown person and assume they were born on the calendar day they tell us; however, by the time they are born, they have already lived through so many experiences in utero which seem to have affected them so much. Where are these experiences stored? And again, Bion does not offer these notions as a developmental theory of the personality, but rather as a way of urging us to suspend a precocious understanding, leaning on our past knowledge of the patient, of their analysis or our theoretical knowledge, when in fact this could be something coming from a completely different world of experience. The grown person may be responding to experiences from far, far away, "*which may even be pre-natal, or pre-birth of a psyche or a mental life*" (Bion, 1977/1989, p. 54).

The caesura of birth is therefore, as already mentioned, a metaphor for all those experiences beyond our capacity to know about or to observe; of course, this was written in 1977, way before ultrasound scans were as popular, apparently revealing so much of intrauterine life.

What are we to think about the patient who does not want to lie on the couch? Is it possible that lying on a couch subjects them to physical pressures of a kind which are beyond their capacity to tolerate, or to verbalize, or to 'understand'?

(Bion, 1977/1989, p. 44)

Again, *just as a model*, say a patient refuses to lie on the couch. We might interpret a resistance, fear of erotic feelings, fear of losing control, and so on and on. We have any number of interpretations derived from adult experience. However, do we really have any idea why that person doesn't lie on the couch? Could it be that, while lying on the couch, there is a dazzling light coming into their eyes, perhaps evoking some prenatal sights, scenes from different worlds, reminiscent of some unbearable intrauterine life? Could we again imaginatively speculate these might be scenes from a time when the amniotic fluid exerted pressure on the eyelids, generating shapes or colors that were excessive, unbearable or overwhelming for the fetus? Can we speculate that lying on the couch is intolerable because it evokes primal, intolerable experiences? Bion again cautions against making interpretations extrapolated from adult experience which we *do* know. And, once more, I would like to reiterate that is but *a model* for experiences that arrive from other universes of experience, incomprehensible, hidden by the impressive caesura created by adult experience. Could we suspend our interpretations so as to get in touch with a different logic than that of our rational, conscious, waking-life logic?

Getting in touch with the ultimate reality of the session requires what Freud denotes as a formal regression of thought, namely from secondary thinking to more primary thinking; not only from Unconscious to Conscious, but also from a more conscious state of mind to one which is unconscious, evoking a quasi-hallucinatory state of mind. We should, as Bion says, be able to give our imagination the freedom to flourish – never mind how ridiculous it might be. And yet, as he reiterates, there are limits. It cannot be an undisciplined, rhapsodical display of just saying anything that comes to our mind. Our imagination, Bion adds, cannot be allowed to develop into an imaginative orgy. He talks about "*analytically trained* intuition", not wild analysis.

This, then, is another vertex from which we can relate to the notion of caesura: the realization that approaching *the patient's* logic requires the analyst to penetrate, or transcend, the caesura of *their* logic, or the logic of the conscious, finite, awake mind, and give their imagination an airing – so as to encounter a different logic, seemingly irrational, or perhaps 'anti-rational'.

We now come to the final vertex from which I would like to approach this paper, namely that of working in the immediacy of the here and now with the prospect of expanding one's capacity to tolerate contact with reality in transit, in the unfolding present. Bion writes:

> Since analysis takes place in time, the tendency is to believe that when the patient is talking he is describing a state of affairs that is also 'ordered' in time; patient and analyst are liable to think of something as having happened in the past. This obscures the fact that we exist in the present; we can do nothing about the past. It is, therefore, seriously misleading to think as if we dealt with the past. What makes the venture of analysis difficult is that one constantly changing personality talks to another.
>
> (Bion, 1977/1989, p. 47)

We are in the habit very often of talking about past events, saying "you probably felt such and such when you were an infant or as a child ... and so on." That seems to be extremely deceptive because, in fact, all that we really know, or all the patient really knows, is what they feel now in the present (Bion, 1975/1991, in Aguayo, 2013).

Bion is highlighting here, as throughout the paper, the necessity of working, of living, in the immediacy of the present. And this present is *in continuous movement towards the future*, requiring us to tolerate being in a state of suspension, entailing suffering.

And why is it so important for us to live in this present? To work in the here and now?

Bion is firmly grounded in Freud's paper on the two principles of mental functioning, and the dialectic movement between the pleasure–pain principle and the reality principle. Bion is aware that being in touch with reality *in transit* is very unsettling and painful. It is painful and intolerable for the mere fact that it is complex, infinite, unpredictable and unknowable in its entirety. That is very difficult and frustrating for us to be in touch with, beyond any painful *content* of reality. So, defensively, we collapse to speaking of reality in static terms, *as if* we were able to know what reality is. Moreover, the narrative of *the events* of reality, ordered in time, affords an illusion of causation. However, that may in fact be a distortion of reality, since we then give way to a one-, two- or three-dimensional apprehension of reality, whereas reality is ever more complex and of *infinite* dimensions. Our tendency to simplify reality amounts to turning away from reality, and that is why Bion talks of psychotic functioning.

Now, Bion is trying to say that what is most difficult for the patient, and for us, is to be in touch with the evolving, perpetually unfolding present. And yet, expanding the patient's ability to be in closer contact with the ultimate reality of the session, in the here and now, might further facilitate the individual's capacity to bear the fact of the reality principle. So, working in the here and now is not only with the objective of repeating, remembering and working through, or in order to uncover early memories or unconscious material, as we often conceive in classical psychoanalytic thinking. No doubt Freud did speak of the past being repeated in the present; Bion does not dispute that. However, here, in this paper, Bion stresses the development of the mind's capacity to tolerate awareness of reality in transit, in the evolving present.

Following the paragraph we have just read, the patient may talk about something that occurred yesterday, or many years ago. Bion never contests the truthfulness of that. However, he *is* asking what *use* the patient is making of this association *now*, in the present? Why are they bringing it up at this specific moment? Is it possible that that is their way of expressing an as yet unmentalized emotional experience they are subjected to in the immediacy of the analytic session right now? The patient may arrive at the session shaken by an accident they had witnessed on the way, but the narrative of the accident itself is so impressive that it may conceal the fact that this serves as a way of *also*, not only, communicating the patient's emotional experience in the immediacy of the session. Is it possible for us not to be so captivated by the past that it creates an impenetrable caesura with the present?

That is very challenging on account of the difficulty to articulate or make sense of the complexity occurring in the present, and, hence, it may be easier to talk to the patient about what happened to them in infancy, or in external reality, even if it might nevertheless also be true. However, we are then in contact with the *repressed* unconscious alone, that which can be symbolically expressed. We are avoiding contact with the unsettling, elusive, ultimate reality of the session, which Bion denotes as O, and with the unconscious which is *not* repressed but nevertheless present right there, in the room. Moreover, as Bion says, "what makes the venture of analysis difficult is that one constantly changing personality talks to another" – that is to say, the fact that the present is in perpetual movement and changing! The minute we talk about it – it's already gone. The interpretation itself, as Bion (1967/2013) says, is very quickly of no further consequence because the interpretation just immediately alters the whole position, and we are confronted again by an unknown situation!

The significant work, then, is not only the meaning the patient might have acquired, but *learning from the experience of tolerating the process and struggle towards a truthful apprehension of reality*, namely, reality in transit, always oriented towards the unknown. That is extremely frustrating, since we all want to get a hold on something substantial that gives us a sense of security.

Bion goes on to say:

> I do not wish to abandon the idea of the conscious or unconscious; the existing theories are valuable, when properly used, either for thinking about a situation or for illuminating the situation for the sake of someone not-self.
>
> (Bion, 1977/1989, p. 47)

Bion still wants to refer to the notion of conscious and unconscious. But he seems to want to take us further.

> These ideas that we hear in the course of analysis have at some time been interpretations though now free associations. We are dealing with a series of skins which have been epidermis or conscious, but are now 'free associations'.
>
> (Bion, 1977/1989, p. 47)

Reality may be likened to the skins of an onion. We can remain in contact with the outermost layers, the epidermis, the conscious, but Bion asks whether we can use these as free associations *on the way* to something concealed, and not as a factual narrative. Just as in dreams we use the day's residues in order to form a dream-narrative, so does the individual use their 'life's residues', or day's residues, in order to form the dream-narrative of that specific session. They may thus articulate their current, as yet unmentalized or unconscious, experience with the aid of the day's residues which they bring from outside the session, just like the infant or the child has to put up with in dealing with quite real things – real experiences – but which cannot be expressed beyond by saying, "I feel I've got a tummy ache". That is the kind of vocabulary, those are the sensuous terms which have to be employed in order to describe a thing which is in no way represented by that at all.

(Bion, 1965/2018)

Moreover, the words only serve as a vehicle for carrying the unmentalized emotional experience. We must not be deluded into thinking that that is what they are actually talking *about*.

So, it is not arriving at some ultimate meaning, but, rather, Bion seems to move us away from the habitual relatedness in classical psychoanalysis – that is to say, between unconscious and conscious – to the movement between finite and infinite, from static to dynamic, towards becoming infinite. Bion is encouraging us to be able to move and observe reality from ever more vertices, always aware that, no matter how much we move towards infinitude, the distance will always remain infinite. Can we be in perpetual movement and observe reality (internal *and* external, sensuous *and* psychic, conscious *and* unconscious, and so on) from forever different perspectives? Ultimately, that would afford a more truthful apprehension of reality, as well as imbuing our emotional experience with psychic aliveness, contrary to calcification in psychic deadness. For Bion, it is not knowing more about reality but rather *being alive in reality*. Stories from the past, and desires for the future, are so impressive that they blind us to what lies beyond, or rather, very often, what lies unobserved right before our eyes. Can we find a way to move beyond that caesura, to find the continuity and be able to encounter more and more meanings?

Bion is concerned with those unsaturated pre-conceptions (with a hyphen) in search of further meanings, rather than saturated preconceptions (without a hyphen).

He further asks whether we might imagine the psychoanalytic session as a game of 'snakes and ladders'. Could we, then, not only strive to arrive at the 100 mark, but rather appreciate the movement? We could throw the dice and land on the 80 mark, almost at the finish, thinking that was a good throw, but then, the following throw, we might move two squares up and roll back down a snake. Was arriving at the 80 mark, then, good or bad? No movement is good or bad in itself but is part of the psyche's movement in the stream of life. Any free association, or any interpretation, is thus neither good nor bad. *It is meaningful.* We must be cautious of the tendency to collapse to a moral outlook, namely 'good' and 'bad', which pertains to psychotic functioning, simplifying and distorting reality. Can we follow the moment-to-moment evolution and try to observe why, where and how we move in the immediacy of the reality of the session? What had the patient, or analyst, responded to? And this is what the analyst should interpret: the evolution.

Bion goes on to say:

> In analysis it is recovery from the unfortunate decision, the use of the mistaken decision that we have to accustom ourselves to deal with. In this view of the position there is no question of a cure.
>
> (Bion, 1977/1989, p. 50)

It is not a 'cure' that the analyst strives for, not the goal of being a well-functioning neurotic, but rather extending one's capacity for movement and for generating meaning – that is, for being psychically alive. Bion always warns us against a 'thus far and no further' attitude. When encountering any circumstance in reality, can we avoid getting stuck, defensively, in deadening repetition and move on? Would it be a break after which we cannot move any further, or will it be a caesura, a break after which there is continuity? In fact, Bion writes that

> 'progress' will be measured by the increased number and variety of moods, ideas and attitudes seen in any given session. There will be less clogging of the sessions by the repetition of material which should have disappeared and, consequently, a quickened tempo within each session every session.
>
> (Bion, 1967/2013, p. 137)

Bion never ceases to stress the ability for motion (e-motion) as a primary criterion for contact with reality. Reality is always in transit, like the river of Heraclitus. The question, then, is how to be in touch with this reality which is in perpetual movement. It is thus the capacity for apprehending reality in transit that is at stake. Not the apprehension of the unconscious, but apprehending its evolution.

Bion's writings are, for me, mostly about *the analyst* and their mind, not only about the patient. The psychotic patient often serves for talking about the analyst when they collapse to psychotic functioning. We all fall into the trap of giving an interpretation which very often becomes a hallucination. We grasp onto some understanding we have at last managed to articulate and we find it hard to let go. We often cannot tolerate our ignorance long enough and thus bring it to a precocious end with a hallucinatory meaning, "that is to say, artificially produced – [a] container intended to hold in, imprison, inoculate the emotional experience the personality feels too feeble to contain without danger of rupture, and so to serve as a vehicle for the evacuatory process" (Bion, 1959/1992, p. 67).

This, of course, touches on another crucial question Bion brings up in this paper, as well as in many others – that of communication. How are we to communicate our intuitions? How do we find a way to convey this to the patient? To our colleagues?

Elsewhere, Bion (1965/1984) writes that he is aware that he too, in writing, falls into the same predicament of using words in order to talk in a deceiving narrative, often implying causation, about something which is complex and ineffable. Yet, he says he hopes that he is using these statements just for the sake of his exposition, keeping in mind that his conceptualizations are fallacious by definition. Psychotic functioning, on the other hand, would be to have certainty that these words are exactly as they say, that they are as they are. We use words and interpretations since they are essential to communication and yet, at the same time, we must not forget their potential for serving as paramnesias, invented to fill the gaps of our ignorance, words used in order to falsely describe something which is ultimately unsayable. "Sometimes", as Bion writes, "the function of speech is to communicate experience to another; sometimes it is to miscommunicate experience to another" (1970/1984, p. 1). In a similar vein, Bion adds, at the end of this paper, that if we use this idea of the caesura between intrauterine life and postnatal life in a concrete or saturated way, it, too, may become static and consequently more of an obstacle than a helpful asset.

Bion is imploring that we remain *in* the caesura, despite the emotional storm and overwhelming aliveness it evokes. Artists can perhaps capture some truthful apprehension of reality encompassing the turbulence of the caesura more than anyone else. For me, it is always reminiscent of Michelangelo's painting on the ceiling of the Sistine Chapel and his intuition of the notion of caesura. We see the finger of God and the finger of Man almost touching, but still retaining the caesura between them. We are captivated by the electricity between these two fingers, which *almost* touch one another, and yet do not. It is because of that small gap that we cannot take our eyes off it. It holds some essential truth that we crave to apprehend. If Michelangelo would have painted the fingers touching each other, we would probably look at it once and perhaps forget it. The fact of this caesura, and the sensuously invisible, alive movement in between, seems to be what accounts for the fact that we are bewitched and cannot let go of it. But that may also be very disconcerting, because we are compelled to tolerate the turbulence evoked by this gap. These are the gap and turbulence Bion is asking us to be in.

References

Aguayo, J. (2013). Wilfred Bion's "Caesura". In H.B. Levine & L.J. Brown (Eds.), *Growth and Turbulence in the Container/Contained: Bion's Continuing Legacy* (pp. 55–74). London: Routledge.

Bion, W.R. (1959 [1992]). Dream-work-α. In *Cogitations* (pp. 62–68). London: Karnac.

Bion, W.R. (1962 [1967]). A theory of thinking. In *Second Thoughts: Selected Papers on Psycho-Analysis* (pp. 110–119). London: Karnac.

Bion, W.R. (1965 [1984]). *Transformations.* London: Karnac.

Bion, W.R. (1965 [2018]). Memory and desire. In C. Mawson (Ed.), *Three Papers of WR Bion* (p. 6). London: Karnac.

Bion, W.R. (1967 [2013]). *Wilfred Bion: Los Angeles Seminars and Supervision.* J. Aguayo & B. Malin (Eds.). London: Karnac.

Bion, W.R. (1970 [1984]). *Attention and Interpretation.* London: Karnac.

Bion, W.R. (1975 [1991]). The dream. In *A Memoir of the Future* (pp. 1–217). London: Karnac.

Bion, W.R. (1976a [1994]). Four discussions. In *Clinical Seminars and Other Works* (pp. 241–292). London: Karnac.

Bion, W.R. (1976b [1994]). On a quotation from Freud. In *Clinical Seminars and Other Works* (pp. 306–311). London: Karnac.

Bion, W.R. (1977 [1989]). Caesura. In *Two Papers: The Grid and Caesura* (pp. 35–56). London: Karnac.

Freud, S. (1926). Inhibitions, symptoms and anxiety. In *Standard Edition*, Vol. 20, pp. 75–176.

Chapter 10

Transformations

João Carlos Braga

The present study focuses on the clinical merits of Bion's theory of transformations (1965/1991), particularly those related to the theory's role in expanding the conceptual and operational psychoanalytic fields to include their ontological dimension. My interest in addressing this theory from a clinical perspective is aligned with my psychoanalytic thinking, which I also recognize in several Brazilian colleagues for whom transformations in being or becoming O are the main theoretical and clinical reference.

Some Background on Bion's Theory of Transformations as a Framework for Clinical Discussion

In *Cogitations* (1992), we can identify that, from the 1950s, Bion was striving to create a basis to develop a scientific theory of the mind. His first attempt was his theory of thinking (1961/1962), which he quickly expanded to a theory of knowledge in *Learning from Experience* (1962), *Elements of Psychoanalysis* (1963), and *Transformations* (1965/1991). The theory of transformations was an expansion of his efforts to give form to realizations that he had from his clinical psychoanalytical practice. *Thinking, knowledge*, and *transformations* were the key elements and cornerstones of each of these theories. Like Archimedes, Bion was looking for a reliable fulcrum with which to move the psychic world. The fact that he stopped searching suggests that he became satisfied with *transformations* as the cornerstone for his theory of the mind. That is, he concluded that any psychic element is a transformation of an inner or outer experience. Indeed, the concept of *groups of transformations* offers the basic parameters to organize the different dimensions of the mind recognized by Bion and to cover potential new ones to be discovered – for example, the idea of a primordial mind.

Even before being introduced into psychoanalysis by Bion, the theory of transformations had a long and illustrious scientific history. The origins of this theory date back to the 1800s with the mathematical theories of *groups, transformations*, and *invariants*. Currently, these theories fertilize many different areas of knowledge, from fundamental calculus and crystallization to

DOI: 10.4324/9781032661230-11

sociology and space travel. Bion was acquainted with these theories, as suggested by their similarities to his theory of transformations and by the names he chose for parts of the theory (groups of transformations, invariants, rigid motion transformations, projective transformations). Furthering this hypothesis are books that Bion had in his library with handwritten notes on this subject (Sandler, 2005, 2016).

Transformations, invariants, and *groups of transformations* have a much more pervasive presence in mental functioning than noticeable at first sight, as every psychic element is a transformation of an inner or external experience with reality. From this perspective, transformations could be seen as the *atoms* of the mind. Still, the theory of groups of transformations and invariants remains at bay in psychoanalysis, leaving the impression that analysts are still struggling to reach what Bion had anticipated by introducing this theory into psychoanalysis. Further developments on this matter can emerge from individual clinical experiences prior to becoming conceptual knowledge shared by analytic groups.

Before delving into the clinical use of the theory of transformations, it will be helpful to discuss some general considerations on this subject:

1   The psychoanalytic theory of transformations has triggered a significant inflection in psychoanalytic thinking and clinical practice. In essence, the concepts of *transformations, groups of transformations*, and *invariants* were revealed to be powerful tools to help analysts identify observations in the psychoanalytic session that can be organized in sets of ideas (groups of transformations) according to their different patterns.

2   A crucial point to bear in mind regarding this inflection is that the psychoanalytic theory of groups of transformations is a field theory – that is, a descriptive, observational theory of the interaction between analyst and analysand and not an explanatory theory of mental processing. In fact, it is a theory of functions and patterns of relationships between an individual and the objects – internal or external ones – in the entire field in which he/she is inserted. Bion made this clear when he pointed out that the aim of psychoanalysis is the study of the "totality of relationships which these objects have to other objects" (Bion, 1965/1991, p. 2). In other words, *any psychic manifestation in the psychoanalytic session must be regarded as a transformation of the analytic experience.*

3   As a theory of relationships *between* objects, the theory of transformations does not deal with objects per se. This dynamic is different in structural theories, in which the whole is composed of interdependent structures – for example, the Freudian and Kleinian models of the mind with their total and part objects. From this perspective, *transformations* and *invariants* acquire a central role in the approach to mental functioning, a role previously occupied by representations and interpretations in traditional psychoanalysis. Perhaps the difference between psychoanalytic

structural and field theories can be thought of as analogous to the difference between physics and chemistry.

4   The approach to mental functioning through the theory of transformations brought significant changes to clinical practice. From the perspective of the theory of transformations, any psychic manifestation in the psychoanalytic session is a transformation of the psychoanalytic experience. Thus, *transformations* and *invariants* acquire a central role in identifying forms of mental functioning, replacing the role historically held by *representations* and *interpretations* in psychoanalysis.

5   The psychoanalytic theory of transformations has had a curious fate since proposed by Bion half a century ago. Although this theory is rarely discussed, parts of it have gained intense penetration in clinical practice, changing the way we think about the mind. The nuclear concept of transformations, the importance of hallucinosis, and – especially – the increasing acceptance of the concept of transformations in being or becoming reality (O) have subtly infiltrated psychoanalytic thinking, even among analysts for whom Bion's work is not recognized as the main reference.[1]

6   The proposal of transformations in being or becoming O brings more challenges to the work of the analyst, but not to that of the analysand, as the latter's requirements remain unchanged. This novel approach to mental functioning has urged the creation of new concepts and ways to deal with psychoanalytic experiences. To overcome the clinical challenges imposed by transformations in O, the analyst must become more involved in the interaction with the analysand and accept being exposed to undifferentiated elements that emerge in the psychoanalytic interconnection.

7   Bion never claimed that his ideas were original or revolutionary in psychoanalysis. On the contrary, he expressed, at different moments, that the contributions from Freud and Klein constituted the common ground for his own scientific deductive system in psychoanalysis. He identified even his most accepted and respected theory – the container–contained theory as the base for mental creation – as a development of Klein's theory of projective identification (1963, p. 3). He clearly mentioned in *Transformations* that what he was presenting was an observational theory and not a theory of mental functioning. He said:

I am therefore ignoring here, and throughout the book, any discussion of psycho-analytic theories. I am however concerned with theories of psychoanalytic observation, and the theory of transformations, the application of which I am here illustrating, is one of them.

(Bion, 1965/1991, p. 16)

Bion was adamant about this in Supervision D14 (1973 or 1974):[2]

PARTICIPANT: Do you consider anything that you have written, so far, or done, as an original contribution to psychoanalysis?

BION: I don't know a single one, not one!

PARTICIPANT: Not even your … what seems to me, at least, the most original of all your written books, the theory of transformations. Don't you consider that an original contribution that has …

BION: Not at all.

PARTICIPANT: No?

BION: No! In fact, I've said over and over again, if you read this book, you'll only understand it when you realize that you're perfectly familiar with the experience.

1   The application of the theory of transformations in psychoanalytical practice may be seen as a fundamental turning point in Bion's work. The theory proposed a new approach and model for mental functioning, changing the way that analysts think about their work. In addition to delving deeply into his theories of thinking and knowledge (Bion, 1961/ 1962, 1962, 1963), it also allowed the psychoanalytic inclusion of direct contact with reality as a mental dimension beyond knowledge and offered tools to organize the coexistence of different systems of analytic thinking.

Clinical Use of the Theory of Transformations

Although psychoanalytic theories are "intended […] for use" (Bion, 1961/ 1962, p. 110), and the theory of transformations is not an exception to that, this theory has seldomly been explored for clinical use. Like Bion's Grid, the theory of transformations is a tool to further investigate mental functioning (1965/1991, p. 75). Bion conceived the Grid (1963b/1997) to examine the end products of transformations of psychoanalytic experiences (Tβ) – that is, elements of the differentiated zones of the personality. We could say that he developed the theory of transformations to tackle the origins of psychic elements generated by experiences (Tα) – that is, the mediums and processes that occur in the undifferentiated zone of the personality.[3]

In clinical practice, the analyst can identify the group of transformations that is present at each movement in the psychoanalytic session. With this aim, I propose to follow Bion's suggestions, taking the Grid as a model and constructing a *table of groups of transformations* as a method to identify and categorize the elements (transformations and invariants) present in the psychoanalytic session:

The grid is intended to remind the psycho-analyst that it is necessary to discriminate one element in his psycho-analytic experience from another and, in particular, to recognize that what matters is both the communication and the use to which it is being put.

(Bion, 1970/1993, p. 4)

It's useful, therefore, to have at your disposal your own particular framework, your own psychological architectonic, so that if you are trying to portray the mind with which you are in contact, you can date various parts of it according to an already prepared schema, a grid of your own construction.

(Bion, 1978/1980, p. 112)

With these data, analysts can be better situated on the different dimensions of the mind at each analytic experience, improving their awareness of the analysand's mental functioning, deepening observations, and gathering elements to reflect on their work.

A Table of Groups of Transformations

If we rely on Bion's thinking to identify the different patterns of transformations in *Transformations* (Bion, 1965/1991), we find two intertwining lines in the description of the groups of transformations. The first relates to the classification of the groups of transformations according to the medium in which the process of transformation occurs (Tα), and the second relates to the final result of each cycle of transformation (Tβ). In the first case, in which the classification is based on the transformation medium, Bion pointed out four patterns in the groups of transformations – namely, transformations in knowledge (K), minus knowledge (–K), hallucinosis, and being or becoming O. The second case, the end product of a transformation cycle, Bion named rigid motion transformations, projective transformations, transformations in hallucinosis, transformations in being O, and transformations in psychoanalysis. In this classification, transformations in hallucinosis and transformations in being or becoming reality appear in both groups as mediums for the processes of transformations (Tα) and, at the same time, as the end product of a transformational cycle (Tβ).

Each of these groups of transformations and invariants gathers specific patterns of mental manifestations comprising observations of different forms of mental functioning. The specificities of the mediums and processes of transformations (Tα) are the factors that determine the end result (Tβ) of each cycle of transformation.

The table of transformations is useful to organize an overview of the distinct groups of transformations for clinical purposes and is open to accommodate new additions and changes. The table summarizes the different groups of transformations, focusing on the four groups that Bion delineated as relying on the mediums and processes of transformations: transformations in knowledge, minus knowledge, hallucinosis, and being or becoming reality (O). To these four groups, I propose the addition of a fifth one to include Bion's ideas on the primordial mind, which he developed between 1976 and 1979, about 10 years after publishing the theory of groups of transformations.

Three groups of transformations have not been included directly in the table – that is, rigid motion transformations, projective transformations, and transformations in psychoanalysis. However, these types of transformations are part of the four groups chosen for the table since their processes of transformations occur in one of the mediums privileged for this classification. For example, transformations in rigid motion (Freudian transformations) are part of transformations in knowledge. For projective transformations (Kleinian transformations), their end products are divided across the different mediums that they go through – that is, (1) elements identified as forms of primitive thinking processes (therefore included in transformations in knowledge); (2) processes of discharging intolerable elements from the mind (i.e., transformations in minus knowledge); and (3) transformations that unburden the mind of intolerable elements but keep sufficient contact with reality to cover with false thoughts the undifferentiated aspect of the psychic reality (hallucinosis evolving as the end results of transformations in a hallucinatory milieu). Finally, transformations in psychoanalysis are part of the set formed by the conjunction of transformations in knowledge and transformations in being or becoming O, the groups of transformations involved with the development of the mind in a psychoanalytic process.

Comments on the Psychoanalytic Table of Groups of Transformations

Comment 1

This table of groups of transformations organizes in rows and columns the analyst's observations of the different patterns of groups of transformations. In a general approach, the table privileges the identification of feelings, emotional processes, and emotional states intuited by the analyst. These identified elements evolve from the analyst's and the analysand's minds, as well as from the interconnection between them.

The rows in the table emphasize three different perspectives:

1   The analyst's general impressions of the session, identifying (a) the emotional, cognitive, and oneiric fluidity; (b) the relationship between the analyst's O and the analysand's O; (c) the transformation medium in which the process occurs; (d) the end result of the transformational cycle; and (e) the prevalent positive or negative emotional link: love, hatred, or knowledge.

	Transformations in Knowledge (K)	*Transformations in Minus Knowledge (−K)*	*Transformations in Hallucinosis*	*Transformations in Being or Becoming O*	*Absence of Transformations (Primordial Mind)*
Analyst's Impressions of the Session (O, Tα, Tβ) + (L, H, K)					
ECO fluidity	• High	• Lowest	• Low	• Highest	• None
Oa / Op	• Convergent	• Very divergent	• Divergent	• Same	• Op not accessible
T medium (Tα)	• K space (containment)	• −K space (projective id, acting-out)	• Hallucinosis	• Being at one	• Body (ANS)
T end result (Tβ)	• Thoughts of the thinker (verbal and oneiric)	• "Without-ness"	• False thoughts (psychic non-reality)	• At-one-ment, atone-ment, at one with O	• Non-integrated psychic manifestations
Links	• +K, +L, +H	• −K, −L, −H	• +/−K, L, H	• Commensal	• Absent
Analyst's Impressions of Own Inner/Otherexperiences in the Session					
Emotional experiences	• Reverie (alpha function, elaboration of EE of the duo) • Interest, vitality, understanding	• Dispersion, devitalization, distraction, disconnection • Somnolence, degrees of stupor • Frustration, irritation	• Emotional mobilization • Enticement • Invitation to not think • Excessive emotions and verbalizations	• To become oneself • Intuitive listening • Constant conjunctions • Negative capability • Enchantment, admiration	• Emptying of intuitions and EE • Somnolence • Anxiety about the lack of contact (autistic states) • Appeal for meanings and reassurance Strangeness, tension
Clinical observations	• Emergence of selected facts • Floating attention • Creation/growth of meanings (thoughts of the thinker)	• Inhibition of the analytical function (EE, intuition, reverie) Negative hallucinations, decathexes, effacement	• Theories instead of experiences • Hallucinosis shared by analyst/analysand	• No search for coherence • Doubts, spontaneity • EE sharing	• Basic, unfounded guilt • Strangeness and terror with emanations from the psyche

Analyst's Impressions of the Analysand's Mental Functioning	Transformations in Knowledge (K)	Transformations in Minus Knowledge (−K)	Transformations in Hallucinosis	Transformations in Being or Becoming O	Absence of Transformations (Primordial Mind)
Verbal communication	• Verbal communication of inner experiences • Free association	• Stripping (−) and reification of meanings • Language as discharge • Lack of attention to the present experience • Deconstruction	• Twisted verbal communication • Hyperbole • Language of substitution	• Language of achievement • Integration of knowledge/emotions/Being • Psychoanalytic conversation • Imaginative conjectures	• Silent proto-mental states • Infiltration in more developed parts of the personality (bubbles)
Analytic situation	• Respect for the limits of the analyst's self	• Disregard for the limits of the psychoanalyst's self (beta screen) • Lack of differentiation between object and its representations • Insensitiveness, dementalization	• Creation of hallucinatory or delusional world • Omnipotence, omniscience, moralistic judgment • Rivalry, superiority, self-sufficiency	• Catastrophic anxieties • Lively presence • Elaborations of Being's experiences (emotions and feelings)	• Instead of emotions, actions or physical manifestations • Psychic events rooted in the body • Urge to exist, primitive conscience, and being all alone and dependent

Note: "Without-ness" is the notation proposed by Sandler (2005, p. 381) as the "predominant characteristic" of a "minus container/contained" process.

Abbreviations: ECO fluidity: emotional, cognitive, and oneiric fluidity, i.e., the dimensions observed; Oa: O of the analyst; Op: O of the patient; T: transformation; Tα: medium in which the process of transformation is occurring; Tβ: the end product of a cycle of transformation; EE: emotional experience; K space: knowledge space; −K space: minus knowledge or not knowledge space; (−): minus point, the non-existent object, "leaving only the place where it was" (Bion, 1965/1991, p. 111); ANS: autonomic nervous system.

2   The analyst's impressions of his/her inner experiences, identifying his/her emotional experiences, as well as other personal observations.
3   The analyst's impressions of the analysand's mental functioning, identifying the verbal communication and characteristics of how the analysand is living the analytic situation.

The columns in the table, as mentioned before, categorize the elements that constitute each group of transformations.

Comment 2: Transformations in Knowledge (K)

It is useful to keep in mind that, when Bion talks about knowledge, he is referring to the process of getting to know and not to the act of possessing some part of knowledge.

In a loose approximation, we could say that transformations in knowledge cover the domain of the thoughts of the thinker. In Bion's theory of knowledge, these transformations would be represented by alpha function, its creation, and the process of dealing with thoughts. Other concepts would also fit well in this group of transformations in knowledge, including the group of transformations in rigid motion, Freud's concepts of transference, the process of symbolization, and Antonino Ferro's (1999) proposal of transformations in dreams. One form of projective transformation – projective identification as the very beginning of a thought – also occurs under this medium and process of transformations in knowledge.

Clinical Vignette

At the beginning of the session, Lucy makes some associations around an event in which she felt as though she was "falling behind" because a colleague received praise for his performance in a task that involved the entire team, including her. In her eyes, this would put her colleague in a position to be promoted. Lucy recognizes that she had not dedicated effort to that task. While talking about it, she shows some discomfort but no defined emotion. The analyst feels that the situation does not require intervention. His impression was that Lucy was working on the situation by herself, but, faced with a prolonged silence, the analyst points out the following, based on what was occurring to him: what would she do now with these comprehensions that she was having?

During another long silence that follows, an image invades the mind of the analyst: a young person (probably himself in earlier times) has his thigh bitten by a small dinosaur (the size of a big dog), ripping a considerable chunk of muscle. He feels no emotion but observes that the injury caused significant damage and ruptured important blood vessels, requiring medical attention. The analyst is unclear about what to do with this image, as he is unable to fit it into the ongoing experience, but accepts the idea that it has to do with something evolving in the analytic situation. The session continues around the same theme for a longer time, with Lucy mentioning how she is satisfied to "work as little as possible," unlike her colleague, who is very dedicated, and whose performance is recognized.

The image of the "small dinosaur" remains in the analyst's mind. Near the end of the session, from an association by the analysand, the analyst comes up with an idea that seems to fit the image. Lucy mentions a movie character who, embittered and struggling to establish affective relationships, meets someone who, little by little, changes the way he (the character) lives his emotions. Intending to help the analysand approximate her own condition to that of this character, the analyst mentions how this embittered character was probably badly hurt in life. Lucy easily grasps and develops the idea.

Comment 3: Transformations in Minus Knowledge (–K)

Transformations in knowledge (K) and minus knowledge (–K) result from the two most basic psychic movements of an individual interacting with reality – that is, incorporating the experience in the form of knowledge (K) or eliminating the disturbing (proto)thoughts and (proto)feelings from the mind, together with parts of the personality that relate to them. A model that could be used here is that of an infant taking an object into its mouth and either ingesting it or spitting it out.

The concept of transformations in minus knowledge covers experiences of projective transformations where the end product is nullifying something that exists in the person's mind or has the potential to be known. In clinical practice, this pattern can be found in mild to intense forms. No-objects take possession violently of what exists in the K space, the space "in which classical transference manifestations become 'sense-able'" (Bion, 1965/1991, p. 115). Sandler (2005) has named this process "without-ness" and described it as a negativating force.

Clinical Vignette

Cora recounts a decisive event in her life that she has mentioned several times before. Reacting to an observation by the analyst about her unusual fluency and clarity while recounting the event, she becomes furious and disappointed. She initially lingers on her understanding that the analyst is never attentive to what she describes. Her irritation grows and gives way to an intense exercise of cruelty toward the analyst. She disqualifies the analytical work and makes heavy accusations about the analyst deceiving her, accusing analysts of putting on façades while having enormous personal difficulties themselves. Cora suddenly stands up from the couch and leaves the room, slamming the door behind her after announcing that she would send the payment for her sessions. The analyst feels impacted by the situation and powerless to deal with what has just evolved but remains receptive to the experience without feeling that he should mull it over. He feels calm and without the need to elaborate further on what he has experienced.

Before the next session, the analyst receives a voice message from Cora, in which she asks if her time slots are still available. The analyst calls her back and confirms that they are still available. In the session that follows the call, Cora begins with a lengthy explanation, without evident guilt or consideration for the analyst. Her explanations preserve the elements that she had previously formulated with violence: she was right about what she had said. However, contrary to the content of her words, the analyst notices an eroticization of the contact without identifiable sensory elements. Perhaps he is reacting to something in the intonation of her voice. The analyst pays attention and, noticing the persistent impression of eroticization, decides to communicate to Cora the thought that organizes in him. He points out her fear that the analysis is exposing her to contact with feelings of love, which in her view are sexual, forbidden, and imprisoning. Cora becomes surprised and more caustic and irritated but contains herself. Without mentioning what the analyst has just said, she begins to describe strong disappointments that she has previously experienced with her parents, husband, and children. The analyst accepts her move and refrains from examining her violence against him. He is convinced that insisting on interpretations of meanings in states of not knowing is not beneficial. He just points out to her that the pain that she was feeling during the session was old and repetitive. The analyst chooses to wait for a future opportunity in which he will feel confident of the presence of resources in the duo to get closer to what terrified Cora. Intuitively, he feels that this is not the case at that moment.

Comment 4: Transformations in Hallucinosis

In "A Theory of Thinking" (1961), Bion introduced the idea of an intermediary condition between tolerance and intolerance of frustrations, which we can recognize as the germ of the group of transformations in hallucinosis:

> If intolerance of frustration is not so great as to activate the mechanism of evasion and yet is too great to bear dominance of the reality principle, the personality develops omnipotence as a substitute for the mating of the pre-conception, or conception, with the negative realization. This involves the assumption of omniscience as a substitute for learning from experience by aid of thoughts and thinking. There is therefore no psychic activity to discriminate between true and false.
>
> (Bion, 1961, p. 114)

Bion extends these ideas in Chapter 10 of *Transformations*, where he presents hallucinosis also as a medium in which rigid motion and projective transformations are processed.

Clinical Vignette

Clive has a collaborative contact with the analyst and communicates with ease his psychic experiences. In a session, he suddenly becomes more serious and comments, with a more decisive voice, that he had been glued to the news about the disaster happening in the mountain region of Rio de Janeiro, which resulted from the heavy rains and landslides on the slopes of the hills. He says that he has been switching from one TV channel to another to look for the latest news. He comments, "You know, I'm disappointed that it's not worse, that more people aren't dying." The analyst feels surprised and waits. Clive mentions other catastrophes and episodes in his daily life in which he found himself having similar reactions. The analyst spontaneously recalls situations in which Clive exaggerated descriptions, presenting himself as a crazy, evil, and morally disqualified person. The analyst mentions his impression that the subject of Clive's description is new, but the pattern is already known to the duo, and reminds Clive of some of these episodes. He also points out Clive's need to check if the analyst endorses this cruelty that he was committing to himself. Clive becomes surprised and talks about how the analytical work allows him to look at his experiences with a comprehension that he had never had. The analyst feels charmed but remains silent. Clive goes on and reports "cat and mouse" games with his wife: when one approaches, the other runs away. The analyst points out the possibility that Clive is now also "running away" from more direct contact with what they were approaching, after praising him (the analyst) and placing both as allies with a superior understanding. Clive laughs nervously and, after a moment of silence, starts talking seriously about his discomfort in the sessions and his fear of the analyst, which appears to be close to what the analyst had noticed.

Comment 5: Transformations in Being or Becoming O.

At some point while writing *Learning from Experience* and *Elements of Psychoanalysis*, Bion conjectured that humans could probably reach reality directly, dispensing with the intermediation of knowledge. The confident way in which Bion presents this idea in *Transformations* suggests that it was a product of a deep and long elaboration. The ability to reach reality directly depends on the analyst being able to bear a deeper involvement with the analysand's undifferentiated layers of mental functioning – a heavy burden. In this situation, the analysis can unfold without the analyst interpreting symbolic meanings in the psychoanalytic situation. In *Transformations* and other publications over the following years, Bion examined carefully how analysts would benefit from adopting this position of elaborating analytic situations after their own ongoing experience (Rezze, 1995/2021, 2001/2021).

Francesca Bion offered us a glimpse of how Bion reached the ideas that he transmitted in his writings:

> He would sometimes emerge from his study, where he had been deep in thought, struggling with these seemingly intractable problems, looking pale and what I can only describe as "absented." It was alarming until I realized that he had been digging so deep in the nature of the psychotic mind that he had become "at-one" with the patient's experience.
>
> (Bion, 1994)

In clinical practice, this movement expanded the analytic field by creating another path (intuition) for analysts to approach mental processes beyond the traditional path (knowledge). Analysts following the path of intuition must free themselves from the gravitational field of knowledge to fly into unknown dimensions, being receptive to points of convergence between theirs and the analysand's minds. Paradoxically, this more abstract dimension of mental development is reached when the analyst becomes involved with the most basic and undifferentiated aspects of the psychic experience, since emotions and their development in feelings are manifestations of *Being*.

Clinical Vignette

At the first session after the holidays, Ben arrives in a good – even effusive – mood and occupies his time by talking excitedly about his travels, enthusiastically detailing the situations he has experienced. The analyst listens for some time, realizing that he (the analyst) had nothing to say. Ben does not seem to be talking to the analyst; he is just talking. The analyst starts feeling increasingly sad but, despite seeing an opportunity to say something based on this feeling, is reluctant to do so owing to concern that he could be experiencing hostility toward Ben's experience on the grounds that Ben has lived something that he has not and doubts that he could be envious of Ben's experience. After some reflection, the analyst evaluates that his feeling of sadness has to do with something going on in the session and decides to tell Ben that, while his descriptions had the quality of something that seemed very satisfying, he also detected a hint of sadness in the air. Ben suddenly sits on the couch and says, almost screaming: "My father had a heart attack." Agitated, he describes in detail an episode during his trip in which his father required intensive care and his life was at risk.

Comment 6: Absence of Transformations (Primordial Mind)

In his striving to approach the origin (O) of the experiences undergoing transformation, Bion was possibly struck at a certain point by a thought that captured his interest over the last years of his life and once more expanded his psychoanalytic view of the mind. The conceptual thought that gave form to this novel idea was the presence in the developed mind of remnants of pre-natal psychic activity, akin to embryonic tissues that remain after birth. According to Bion's conjecture, these elements indicated the possible existence of a primordial mind, in contrast with the Kleinian primitive mind and the Freudian symbolic mind, which develop after birth in the context of object relationships. Over the last 3 years of his life (1976–1979), Bion investigated and elaborated imaginative and rational conjectures on this very beginning of mental life and formulated them empirically and loosely as parts of a pri-mordial mind. He identified three different forms for these manifestations and named them "urge to exist," "being all alone and dependent," and "primitive conscience" (Junqueira de Mattos & Braga, 2009/2013; Braga, 2020). These elements could be considered a fifth group of transformations, characterized by the absence of transformations, and appearing infiltrated in manifestations of the developed mind. Korbivcher studied these conjectured prenatal ele-ments extensively under the umbrella of the theory of transformations and identified two groups of elements, which she named *autistic transformations* (2001/2014) and *non-integrated transformations* (2017).

Clinical Vignette

Avery is very rigid regarding his ability to think. He frowns upon his own thoughts and treats them as dangerous products, often as "very crazy things." He feels comfortable in "thinking" what others "think." The analyst sees Avery as a person with significant resources in terms of sensitivity, curiosity, and intelligence, but without the ability to achieve personal and professional developments that could benefit him. He lives within a small circle, where the elaboration of present experiences is limited. In the analytical work, Avery suffers significantly when in contact with his mental life. He sometimes gives evidence of not recognizing the presence of the analyst and seems to entertain ways not to establish object relationships. He avoids examining what emerges in the psychoanalytic situation. When the analyst presents this to him, he becomes distressed, tries to avoid deepening the examination, and moves away from the topic in focus. At the same time, he has many somatic com-plaints that arise mainly from excessive food intake. It is also meaningful to observe his attachment to certain things: "Why do I always bring this brief-case?" "Why can't I stop smoking?" "Why don't I leave this city?"

In a given session, more than 10 years into Avery's analysis, the analyst is experiencing with him the usual atmosphere of absent emotional contact, while Avery describes his ideas. Avery suddenly interrupts this trend and establishes contact, with surprising fluidity, in which it becomes possible to examine the experience of the session in a remarkably meaningful way. He describes perceptions of himself with great creativity and dreamlike freedom, tolerating ambiguities and duplicities. He shows a capacity to deal with doubts: "It can be like this; it can be like that." When the analyst points out that he (the analyst) now recognizes him (Avery) using conditions to establish contact that he does not usually use, Avery becomes scared and distressed: "But by doing this, I feel like falling apart." The analyst refrains from saying anything, feeling that both he and the analysand are experiencing a significant moment of contact in a frame of mind that is always present, but not necessarily prevalent. In the analyst's experience, his words would be peripherally meaningful in Avery's psychic state.

Final Considerations

Observation I

The proposed table of groups of transformations summarizes the different forms of transformations and helps the analyst identify, at a glance, the ongoing patterns in the session. The table is based on the postulate that each group of transformations binds a proper set of patterns and elements. It also helps the analyst to reflect on specific manifestations happening in the duo – analyst–analysand. As Bion presented:

> The investigation of this and other analytical experiences should in time enable us to see different types of transformation and perhaps to arrive at some classification of the different sets of transformation which together make up the group of transformations.
>
> (1965/1991, p. 14)

Observation 2

In clinical practice, the distinction between groups of transformations is not clear-cut. In some areas, forms of transformations overlap, and the analyst must identify the prevalent one. Also, elements belonging to more than one group of transformations can be conjectured as being present in the same transformation cycle.

In different moments, Bion warned us about this overlapping:

> It is a matter of consequence because the decision depends in what is more convenient for the analyst.

He added in a footnote:

> And the decision the analyst takes is to identify with a particular vertex.
>
> (Bion, 1965/1991, p. 26)

This thought is expanded in Chapter 10:

> Nothing in the practice of psychoanalysis ever fits into neat and rigid categorization.
>
> (Bion, 1965/1991, p. 132)

This is possibly the same issue that we find when we consider Bion's observation about the coexistence of positive and negative links of love, hate, and knowledge (1962, p. 44) or when we interpret a clinical episode through different psychoanalytic lenses.

Notes

1 The present author offers a more extensive discussion of these issues in "Empowered by Failure – Vicissitudes of Transformations", Braga, 2008/2022.
2 I am grateful to José Américo Junqueira de Mattos, who collected, preserved, translated, and made available more than 130 supervisions held by Bion during his four visits to Brazil (1973, 1974, 1975, and 1978). I am also thankful to Gisèle Mattos Brito for providing the original recordings and transcriptions of the supervisions included in this presentation.
3 I am using here "differentiated and undifferentiated zones" of the personality having in mind the integrative model that R. Vermote proposed for the function of the mind after "late Bion's" contributions (Vermote, 2011, 2019).

References

Bion, F. (1994). Personal communication.
Bion, W.R. (1961/1962). A theory of thinking. *International Journal of Psychoanalysis*, 43.
Bion, W.R. (1962). *Learning from experience*. London, William Heinemann.
Bion, W.R.(1963). *Elements of psychoanalysis*. London, William Heinemann.
Bion, W.R. (1963b/1997). The Grid. In: W.R. Bion. *Taming wild thoughts*. F. Bion (Ed.). London, Karnac.
Bion, W.R. (1965/1991). *Transformations*. London, Karnac.
Bion, W.R. (1970/1993). *Attention and interpretation*. London, Karnac Books.
Bion, W.R. (1973 or 1974). Supervision D14. Audiotape of supervision given in Rio de Janeiro. Transcription and notation by José Américo Junqueira de Mattos.
Bion, W.R. (1978/1980). Seminars in São Paulo. In: *Bion in New York and São Paulo*. Perthshire, Clunie Press.
Braga, J.C. (2008/2022). Empowered by failure – vicissitudes of Transformations. In: *Bion's Legacy in São Paulo*. Rezze, C. & Marra, E. (Eds.). London and New York, Routledge.
Braga, J.C.(2020). Developments on the concept of superego in Bion's work. *International Journal of Psychoanalysis*, 101 (4).
Ferro, A. (1999). O Sonho da Vigilia: Teoria e Clínica. *Revista Brasileira Psicanálise*, 33 (3).
Junqueira de Mattos, J.A. & Braga, J.C. (2009/2013). Primitive conscience: A glimpse of the primordial mind. In: Levine, H.L. & Brown, L.J. (Eds.), *Growth and turbulence in the container/contained*. London and New York, Routledge.

Korbivcher, C.F. (2001/2014). The theory of transformations and autistic states. Autistic transformations: a proposal. In: Korbivcher, C.F., *Autistic transformations*. London, Karnac.

Korbivcher, C.F. (2017). Bion and unintegrated states: falling, dissolving and spilling. In: Levine, H. & Power, D. (Eds.), *Engaging primitive anxieties of emerging self*. London, Karnac.

Rezze, C.J. (1995/2021). Estudo de uma sessão analítica: Identificação e rastreamento na clínica dos conceitos de inconsciente, sexualidade, recalcamento, transferência e transformações [Studying an analytic session: clinical identification and trailing of the concepts of unconscious, sexuality, repression, transference and transformations]. In: Rezze, C.J., *Psicanálise: de Bion ao Prazer Autêntico*. São Paulo, Blucher.

Rezze, C.J. (2001/2021). Fantasmas e Psicanálise: Digressão em Torno de Transformações em O [Ghosts and psychoanalysis: Digression around transformations in O]. In: Rezze, C.J., *Psicanálise: de Bion ao Prazer Autêntico*. São Paulo, Blucher.

Sandler, P.C. (2005). *The language of Bion – a dictionary of concepts*. London, Karnac.

Sandler, P.C. (2016). Transformations? Invariants! Presented at Bion's International Meeting, Milan.

Vermote, R. (2011). On the value of "late Bion" to analytic theory and practice. *International Journal of Psychoanalysis*, 92, 1089–1098.

Vermote, R. (2019). *Reading Bion*. London, Routledge.

Chapter 11

Negative Capability

Navigating the Paradox in the Language of
Achievement and the Language of
Substitution

Afsaneh Alisobhani

In the memorial meeting for Dr Wilfred Bion (1981), Francesca Bion wrote beautifully about Bion's love for poetry. She wrote that Bion hoped to compile a book of poetry for psychoanalysts. Unfortunately, he was not able to complete the project, but, in that meeting, Francesca shared what Bion wrote as an introduction for this collection. He wrote:

> I resort to the poets because they seem to me to say something in a way which is beyond my powers and yet to be in a way which I myself would choose if I had the capacity. The unconscious – for want of a better word – seems to show the way "down to descend", its realms have an awe-inspiring quality.
>
> (Bion, 1981)

In 1973, in one of his seminars in New York, Bion asked "what kind of poets and artists can we be as psychoanalysts?" (Bion, 1980, p. 73). It is no wonder that he ends the last chapter of his book, *Attention and Interpretation* (1970), with inspiration from a letter John Keats wrote to his brother and that he titled the chapter "Prelude to or Substitute for Achievement". Since some of you may not be familiar with this writing, allow me to start today's talk by repeating the quote from Keats.

> I had not a dispute but a disquisition with Dilke on various subjects; several things dove-tailed in my mind, and at once it struck me what quality went to form a Man of Achievement, especially in Literature, and which Shakespeare possessed so enormously – I mean Negative Capability, that is when a man is capable of being in uncertainties, mysteries, doubts, without any irritable reaching after fact and reason.
>
> (Keats, 1958, p. 60)

Dilke was a politician who devoted much of his life to the pursuit of literature at that time, and Keats contrasts his words to those of William Shakespeare. What makes Shakespeare's words durable throughout centuries is

DOI: 10.4324/9781032661230-12

his capacity to *observe* the human condition and suffer the pain of not knowing. Having access only to what is real, Shakespeare dared to step in the direction of imagining the truth and speaking to that truth. According to Keats, he was able to do that through his capabilities for negative space – that is, he was able to allow plenty of room for mystery and doubt. Truth, in all its beauty, will almost fortuitously reveal itself. It is the poet in the psychoanalyst, according to Bion, who apprehends and suffers the aesthetic dimensions of this intuitive form of knowing, beauty and the catastrophe of pain juxtaposed with one another.

This revelation is only possible through the language of achievement. Bion believed that the analyst in the consulting room must listen and see everything as if she is reading poetry. As one reads the words, the deeper meaning, the truth, in all its beauty and horror, will reveal itself. It is the emotional experience of both the analyst and the patient that ultimately leads to transformation; Bion called it a transformation from K to O. Language of achievement must possess a quality that is penetrating, permeating time and space, the way Shakespeare's did, persisting through centuries.

Meltzer elaborates on the aesthetic dimension of knowing and being in the presence of the mother's beauty and the conflicting joy and pain that ensue. The resolution of the aesthetic conflict is incumbent upon one's negative capability. Does the infant evade the seemingly unbearable pain and try to escape the agony by resorting to lies and fragmentation? Or allow himself to suffer the pain and navigate the sensorial world and move to imagination? One route is the language of substitution, a language that is already saturated and comes from memory and desire and, therefore, with the need for certainty; the other is the language of achievement. One is anti-growth, it is about falsity, with a quality of –K belonging to column 2 of the grid, while the other makes room for painful experience, and therefore meaning, with the K link in search of truth. Negative capability, the mental space for the language of achievement, "that is both a prelude to action and itself a kind of action; the meeting of psycho-analyst and analysand" (Bion, 1970, p. 125) belongs to the grid category D4. Bion (1965, p. 77) refers to one, the –K view, as "backward-looking and relating to what has been lost" and the other, "the ordinary view as forward-looking and relating to what can be found". The analyst willingly steps into dangerous territory and must be aware and vigilant of this danger while listening to the patient's material. Bion maintains, however, that a psychoanalyst must "watch and listen to a person while he is understanding and while he is misunderstanding" (Bion, 1990, p. 63). In other words, he suggests that, for an analytic encounter to be effective, the analyst must stay sharp and listen for both language of substitution and language of achievement, in both himself and in the patient. He must have what he calls a "binocular vision". In *Transformations* (1965), Bion writes:

Superficially an analytic session may appear boring, or featureless, alarming, or devoid of interest, good or bad. The analyst, seeing beyond the superficial, is aware that he is in the presence of intense emotions; there should be no occasion on which this is not apparent to him.

The intense experience is ineffable but once known cannot be mistaken ...

The approach to it, to be effective, is 'binocular'; the analyst must be aware, while attending to the patient's material, of the dangers of his association with that particular patient: he should be able to see what the danger is that the patient is inviting him by his presence to share.

(pp. 74–75)

Identical words, gestures, or a grunt can be utilized to represent a substitute for action or the language of achievement, a prelude to action. Bion conjectured that some analyses that seemed to be endless may be an example of analyses where the language of substitution is taken as the language of achievement.

So, how is the language of achievement a prelude to action? Conversely, what are the factors leading to the detour to the language of substitution?

Bion invoked the idea of transformation to reconsider psychoanalytic thinking, moving from a static, positivistic stance to one that is in a constant state of flux, from classical physics to quantum mechanics, from Newton to Heisenberg, from particles to waves; in other words, adopting a philosophical and scientific model that reflects real life. He was interested in figuring out the process we adopt when encountering the changing circumstances.

How, in the face of immediacy of life experience, do we metabolize and digest the emerging uncertainties and weather the storm of the inevitable "emotional turbulence"?

The object of this transformational process is what Bion calls 'O'. At this point, I want to take a few minutes to review and describe what I understand Bion means by O. Arnaldo Chuster (2014) describes O as the expansion of Bion's theory of preconception. He sees O as "the solution and the conflict of the human species in his search for survival." He goes on to elaborate on this process from a phylogenetic perspective. The evolutionary process and a relatively short gestational period diminish the influence of the innate and force the human infant to learn from experience. Chuster writes:

pre-human babies were born more and more "unfinished" and their complete maturation occurred after birth through interaction with society. The transmission of knowledge and behavior became more and more important. Thus, the pre-conception can be understood in the first place as a vestige in the mind of the passage of the pre-human to human.

(p. 26)

Following Kant's theory of knowledge, Bion modeled his theory of thinking on this concept. The human infant is born with the preconception of not only his mother's breast, but also her mind behind the breast – what Bion called the mother's capacity for reverie. The process of *finding and experiencing* the breast and meeting the mother's mind sets the stage for the human infant to emotionally learn from the experience of the encounter. This process of *finding and re-finding* helps expand and grow the baby's mind. The mother's capacity for reverie and containment grows to accommodate her baby's emotional needs. It is this continuous cycle of preconception and realization that is responsible for the complexity of the human mind. It is in this vein that Chuster describes Bion's O as an expansion and elaboration of preconception.

Bion borrows from Plato's theory of forms to substantiate his theory of preconception. Chuster (2018) suggests that O stands for both origin and process. O stands for *origin*, "ontos" in Greek, one's emotional response to the raw, sensory experience of an encounter with the internal as well as the external object. As this experience becomes personal and known, what Bion calls a transformation from O to K, a process of learning from experience, starts to develop. James Grotstein uses saliva as a metaphor. He writes "we unconsciously decide – through transformations – to impart our metaphoric 'saliva' of personal-ness onto each input from the other and then claim it as our own" (Grotstein, 2007, p. 213).

'O' also stands for *process*, "opus" in Greek; it is inherently destabilizing, unknown, and unknowable. It is the *process* of learning from experience that brings about wisdom, and wisdom brings about a capacity to think and make connections with internal and external objects. For Bion, O is not unlike the Kantian phenomena – we can only know it by its representation in the process of transformation, and never the thing-in-itself. Grotstein writes "when O is felt to be overwhelming, thus *it* helps the individual stricken by O to 'die a little' emotionally, adaptively, in order to remain alive as a self" (Grotstein, 2007, p. 115). In the analytic situation, as the analyst experiences the O of the session and allows herself to be transformed by the process, she will learn and gain wisdom and knowledge from this experience, hence a transformation from O to K. It is in this space that the analyst, with her newfound knowledge about the patient and herself, can help the patient in his process of maturation and growth (Bion, 1965). For a transformation from K to O to take place, the analyst and patient must be willing to tolerate the darkness, dare to face the danger, for the possibility of a flash of light that illuminates the road – what Bion calls the process of becoming O (Bion, 1965, p. 159). Bion called the process of a transformation from K to O the "psychoanalytic transformation" (Bion, 1965, p. 144).

Depending on whether the psychotic or the non-psychotic part of the personality is dominant, the process of transformation takes on different forms. Since the emotional states of both the patient and analyst are in a state of flux, the process of transformation may take a detour to one of the following types as a means of evading the psychoanalytic transformation.

Rigid Motion Transformation

Rigid motion transformation corresponds to what in classical Freudian analysis is defined as transference neurosis. Infantile wishes and repressed feelings are transferred onto the person of the analyst. It is *rigid* because it hasn't changed in form and shape. It is the predominant process of transformation for the "neurotic character" or the neurotic part of the personality. Clinically, by talking about the past in a clear way, the patient is trying to take the psychoanalyst to that place in the past, as if that place was in the present moment.

Projective Transformation

In contrast to rigid motion transformation, which is modeled on Euclidean geometry, Bion borrowed the concept of projective transformation from projective geometry. It corresponds to the Kleinian concept of projective identification as a form of communication and the experience of being with the patient in the P-S (paranoid-schizoid) position. In projective transformation, the patient's communication is distorted and creates confusion. The patient's verbal communication "is meaningless, but can act as a stimulus to speculation" (Bion, 1965, p. 21).

Transformation in Hallucinosis

Transformation in hallucinosis corresponds to an *emotional state* in the domain of what Bion call "hallucinosis" where a "state of complete freedom from the restriction imposed by contact with realization of any kind" is *seemingly* realized (Bion, 1965, p. 134). As opposed to hallucination, which is sensory, the state of hallucinosis is when an emotional experience is used in the service of hallucinatory gratification instead of making use of it for the development of the mind and development of thought. A state of hallucinosis, under the dominance of the pleasure principle, is free from the restrictions of time and space; it is the domain where thinking and meaning are replaced by moral judgment. In the domain of hallucinosis, ethical gratification[1] is sacrificed for the pleasure imbued in morality. This experience, stripped of meaning, ironically leaves the patient in agony and even more frustrated. He greedily turns to more hallucination to escape the pain, only to face more of it. Bion writes, "the less gratification he achieves the more greedy he becomes☒ the more greedy, the more hallucinated" (Bion, 1970, p. 37). Sandler (2005, p. 782) describes it as an example of "psychosis of everyday life".

To transcend transformation in hallucinosis to transformation in K, the analyst, a participant observer, relies on his own emotional experience for guidance. The psychoanalyst must allow himself to experience the state of hallucinosis as the O of the moment. Bion believed that, when a person is having a transformation from K to O, she is in a state of not knowing; all she can do is tolerate the uncertainty. Language of achievement comes from this transformational process. Bion writes, "Language of Achievement includes language that is both prelude to action and itself a kind of action; the meeting of psychoanalyst and analysand is itself an example of this language" (Bion, 1970, p. 125).

Language of Achievement

John Keats said that a poet has no identity. When he writes poetry, he can take on different characters, depending on what character the poetry calls on him to be in that moment. As he becomes a character, the language comes to the poet, and in a way the poem writes itself. Jim Grotstein used to say that analysts must become Stanislavsky method actors, they must become who the patient needs them to be (Grotstein, 2006). If there is a space for the unknown and the unknowable, both the analyst and analysand become in touch with the O of the session.

In his paper "Language and the Schizophrenic" (1955), Bion links the depressive position with the development of verbal thought and its role in awareness of internal and external reality. Meltzer, however, imagines the agonizing experience of that moment in time to be so unbearable that the baby reverts to the dreaded P-S position. The image of the "ordinary beautiful mother" and the "ordinary beautiful baby" in the depressive position, in awe of the mother's beauty, "against the dazzle of the sunrise", is too painful to bear for the baby. The baby, all too aware (albeit unconsciously) that the mother who giveth can take it away, retreats into his Platonic cave of the paranoid-schizoid position. But, eventually, he emerges from the cave (Meltzer & Harris Williams, 1988). Through learning from the experience of the repeated oscillation between P-S and D and surviving the "catastrophic change" (Bion, 1970, p. 91), "Negative Capability exerts itself, where Beauty and Truth meet" (Meltzer & Harris Williams, 1988, p. 28). Bion viewed observation and patience as the analyst's most valuable instruments in realizing negative capability. He was impressed by Charcot's impact on Freud in advising him to patiently observe his patients until a pattern begins to emerge (Bion, 1976/1994, p. 285).

Clinical Example

The following vignette may help shed some light on the contrasting aspects of language of achievement and the language of substitution. This patient has been in analysis with me, four times a week, for the past two years. John is a 35-year-old gay married man who struggled with his sexuality and relationships. Although married for almost 10 years, he never had sex with his husband – they cuddled and kissed, but that was the extent of it. He never had any extramarital sexual relationships and, prior to marriage, he had very few sexual encounters; he preferred masturbation to engaging sexually with another person. He recently decided to separate from his husband because he felt that, although he loved him deeply and had a strong emotional and intimate relationship with him, he was never in love with him. He never felt the passion his husband felt for him and would never fall in love with him. As a matter of fact, recent developments led him to believe that he had never experienced passionate love for another man. Ironically, he started analysis with me because he fell in love with a coworker and, for the first time, he felt "that fire in his belly". John could no longer deny what was lacking in his marriage. Tom, a fellow investment banker, is heterosexual and has been seemingly happily married for some time. Nonetheless, John, vacillated between wishing that Tom was gay to being certain that he was and that he just didn't know it yet. John's separation from his husband was prompted by his strong feelings for Tom, as he realized what was missing in his life up to that point. What started as casual conversations in the office turned to friendship; sometimes the two would even go to lunch. Their encounters were limited, as they worked on different floors. John's mood, however, hinged on the level and quality of his engagement with Tom on a given day. One day he would come to the session on cloud nine because Tom was warm and friendly toward him; the next day he was devastated and hopeless because Tom ignored him or was friendly with another co-worker.

John is an accomplished young man: he holds multiple degrees, he speaks multiple languages, and he is friendly and likeable. Yet, he doesn't feel secure in his job. He lives in a constant state of flux, vacillating between a feeling of being petrified that he'll lose his job to becoming quite arrogant and entitled, treating his co-workers and manager in a condescending manner. This attitude has gotten him in trouble at work and elsewhere. A similar dynamic occurs in analysis; he is open, committed to analysis, but finds little value in any interpretation I have to offer. A statement from me nudging him to look for the meaning of what he is experiencing, however gentle, evokes either a feeling of shame and persecution or an angry response, accusing me of being cold or just plain wrong. On either occasion, the expression on his face tells another story. It reminds me of a baby suddenly awakened by a loud noise, looking startled and disoriented. It is heartbreaking to watch him flinch, physically trying to get rid of the deep-seated, amorphous fear. Defensively, he immediately adopts an arrogant posture and tells me that I am wrong, all he wants from me is validation and I keep questioning him. His arrogance toward me, however, feels hollow. It feels like a petrified little boy who is trying to act brave and puff himself up, letting me know that he is a man and not being swallowed by his fears. Confused, I have been talking less and less, trying to observe and listen more intently, not just to what he shares verbally, but also to his body language, his penetrating stare, and his rare silent pauses. He talks a great deal, he cries, he screams, yet I have a hard time connecting to his affects. I feel like I am watching an amateur play, with an amateur actor. Sessions are filled with what Tom did or didn't do that day. I often wonder why he keeps coming to analysis, as he tells me that, when he recounts the same stories to his friends, they always have something more empathetic or profound to tell him.

There is something else that happens in the analysis that I feel is significant. After I meet him in the waiting room, as he walks into the consulting room, he always makes a comment about my appearance. He says something about my clothes, my hair, my makeup, always complimentary and polite. As soon as he sits on the couch, he stares right into my eyes, and it feels as if he is piercing my skull, leaving very little space for me to think. He tried to lie on the couch, but the experience was too disturbing for him, he had a visceral reaction to it. The heightened anxiety was palpable. Needless to say, there is no room for interpretation. I used to be really annoyed with his comments about my appearance. They were not necessarily intrusive – it felt more like he was de-emphasizing our professional relationship and treating me like I was an aunt or a family friend. At best, we were cuddling – there was not much room for intercourse. I also felt a sense of rivalry, a jockeying for position from him. It didn't feel like he was trying to control me, but more like he needed to declaw and defang me. It worked! I really wasn't sure what to do with that. Intuitively, I knew interpreting the rivalry or even his attempt at protecting himself from me was just the tip of the iceberg. Lately, I have started to see a different side to the ritual, a different feeling emerged in me. I imagined the "ordinary beautiful baby" allowing himself to meet "the ordinary beautiful mother", and the aesthetic conflict that Meltzer wrote about ensued. The depressive anxieties, however, quickly turned to the violent emotions in the P-S position; John couldn't stay in that space to allow for any meaning to emerge. Instead, he would quickly erase her/me as soon as he sat on the couch and vigilantly stared into my eyes. I was able to feel his agonizing pain, always on the lookout, ready to fight, yet he looked so hungry, hoping for something magical from me to make it all go away.

On one day, I was returning from a trip to Catalina Island. Before getting on the ship, I stopped at a souvenir shop at the port, and my eyes caught this notebook. There was a sketch of a mermaid on the cover with a saying, "Kinda pissed for not being a mermaid". I thought it was silly, but I bought it for my daughter for a quick laugh. When I went to the office the next day, the notebook was still in my purse, I forgot to give it to her. When John arrived (he was the sixth or seventh patient of the day), before I went to greet him, I mindlessly went through my purse, reached inside, and grabbed the notebook. Habitually, if I have a book I am reading, I either remove it from sight or leave it face down. Since John usually scans the room and makes a comment if there is anything different in the room, I try to be extra careful not to leave anything around to arouse curiosity. On this day, however, I inadvertently left the notebook face up. John noticed the cover and read it out loud, "Kinda pissed for not being a mermaid". I felt embarrassed, foolish, and a little exposed. I had this urge to say something to divert his attention (language of substitution) but held back and tried to stay present with him. Being quite well schooled in all kinds of mythology, he didn't miss a beat and, as soon as he sat down, he asked me if I knew the origin of the mermaid story. A little relieved that he was going into *his* language of substitution, I said, no. He said that this Assyrian goddess fell in love with a mortal shepherd and unintentionally killed him; she felt so ashamed that she jumped into the sea to become a fish so she would never have to face another human being. But the ocean wouldn't conceal her godlike beauty, turning her into a mermaid, half fish, half human. At this point, a profound sense of sadness came over me. I felt it had something to do with him, but I couldn't quite formulate a thought or utter a word. Without missing a beat, he shifted gear and went on to tell me about his problems at work; he was worried that he would not be promoted, since his boss gave him some negative feedback. It was interesting that his boss, an accountant, told him that he lacked *self-awareness*. John said, "it was deflating, as you'd like to put it, Afsaneh! ... it is funny that word, deflating, like deflating a balloon". I was surprised that he actually took in something I said. I wasn't sure if he remembered the word because of its impact on him, or he liked the music and cadence of the word itself. He then went on to tell me that he made an elaborate flow chart with all possible options at work. He showed me the chart; it was a jumble of lines and circles, emblematic of the emotional space he lived in most of the time. He said, "I am trying to game everything through to get promoted". He went through different scenarios of what he could do to move up the ladder at work, ignoring his boss's revealing comment. He abruptly changed course again and said, "Or should I come right out, put everything on the line and come out to Tom and tell him that I am in love with him and I think he is in love with me?" He continued that, if it weren't for his secret crush on Tom, he would've left this job a long time ago. He raised his voice in anger and said that he was way too overqualified for the position; they were not paying enough for him to work with such incompetent people. His affect quickly shifted to a pensive place; I felt a sense of sadness in him, what I had been feeling a moment earlier when he was telling me the mermaid story. The moment was quickly lost; he shifted in his seat, cleared his throat, resigned, and said *"well, what are you going to do?"* Bion would say he was back in column 2 territory. Yet, I could tell that he was really scared to lose his job; he couldn't take the humiliation of being let go. Still unclear about who Tom really was to him, I nonetheless thought that the idea of never seeing Tom again felt to John like the air was being sucked out of his lungs. I remembered that, when he first came to analysis, he told me that he had this irrational fear of becoming homeless. We sat quietly for a few minutes (quite unusual for him). After a few minutes, he had a smile on his face, he said, "but yesterday *Tom was so cute*, I think he was flirting with me". Then suddenly, he said, "oh my god, I almost forgot to tell you! I had this dream last night". He proceeded to share a dream. In the dream, he went to a doctor who specialized in euthanasia. John wanted to be put to death. The doctor asked him if he was sure he wanted to go through with it. "I said yes", he responded. The doctor told him, "We just puncture your lung, you die of suffocation, but you won't feel anything". John continued,

> He punctured my lung, it was really surreal. I could see my lung with the hole in it. I *did* feel the pain, I felt like I was gasping for air, suffocating. It was scary, I panicked, oh my god, oh my god, I can't breathe. I woke up in a sweat but then I started crying [he started crying as he was talking]. I had this horrible thought that even if Tom accepts my proposition, even if he tells me he's gay, even if we start to go out with each other, what's going to happen? I don't know what I'll do. I don't know if this will be a good thing for him. That'll bring so much turmoil and instability for him, I don't want him to go through that! Even worse, what if he decides not to leaves his wife? What if he tells me this was all my imagination? What if he says he's not gay?

We were getting toward the end of the hour. There was so much in this dream, yet I couldn't utter a word. We were quiet, but, in a moment of lucidity, as if my lips had a mind of their own, I said "You're really scared, aren't you? You are scared that *you are the mermaid*". In a surprising move, he made a fist with his hand and hit his chest, as if puncturing his own lungs, instead of rejecting my interpretation outright. He said, "That's always been my deepest, darkest secret, that I was never really meant to be with anyone. But I could never put it into words." He cried quietly for the rest of the session and, as he was leaving, he said "Weird ... I feel so much lighter ... huh!"

Bion describes the state of hallucinosis as a state where the "disturbed patient" is "conscious of a 'past' that no longer exists" and the analyst "to be Unconscious of a 'future' that has not come to pass" (Bion, 1965, p. 85) – *avant coup* as opposed to *après coup*. He further argued that, to help a patient in making the transformation from K to O, the analyst must be open to participate in hallucinosis with the patient and be able to step back and tolerate the uncertainty. It is only in this negative space that a new word might come to the analyst and help the patient with transformation. I feel that I momentarily joined John in a state of hallucinosis as I unconsciously moved to the "future" that had not yet occurred when I mindlessly brought the notebook to the consulting room. Subsequently, as an analytic couple, we were both able to discover a new word, *mermaid*!

In retrospect, I thought about the story of Odysseus and his travails, as he tried to return to Ithaca after the Trojan War. He traveled with the mermaids with hypnotic singing voices. They lured sailors into the depths of the sea, to their death. To protect himself and his sailors from them, Odysseus asked his sailors to plug their own ears so that they wouldn't hear the mermaids sing and then tie him to the mast, so that he wouldn't be seduced by the enchanting voices of the mermaids. Once they had traveled out of earshot, the sailors were to untie him. Some versions of the myth state that, if anyone escapes the mermaids, the mermaids will drown themselves and die.

Most of the time, in a state of hallucinosis, John ties himself to the mast, turning a deaf ear to my interpretations, protecting himself from my voice, which might otherwise seduce him to the depths of his unconscious.

But I, in my own state of hallucinosis, survived the mermaid/John/Odysseus hypnotic voice/evasion and lived to sail/sing another day. Bion believed that negative capability is within the reach of "all of us ordinary analysts", as he stated in one of his lectures in São Paulo:

> Keats said that Shakespeare must have been able to tolerate mysteries, half-truths, evasions, in order to be able to write. He had to be able to pay the price if he wanted to be Shakespeare. What he wrote still endures; it has a toughness, durability which we cannot achieve; and yet he was an ordinary person like the rest of us. What makes people like Shakespeare and Virgil and Milton so "extraordinary" is their ability to do such extraordinary things while at the same time being ordinary. All of us ordinary people must dare to behave as if we were extraordinary without believing that it is the case, without being cheats.
>
> (Bion, 1990, p. 46)

Note

1 Arnaldo Chuster describes ethical gratification as a sequence of events that begin with sincerity. Sincerity, in turn, brings words of honor that help create a character capable of courage, compassion, and respect for truth. (Personal Communication, 2019)

References

Bion, F. (1981) Memorial Meeting for Dr. Wilfred Bion. *International Review of Psychoanalysis*, 8: 3–14.

Bion, W.R. (1955). Language and the Schizophrenic. In M. Klein, P. Heimann, & R. E. Money-Kyrle (Eds.), *New Directions in Psychoanalysis* (pp. 220–239). London: Karnac.

Bion, W.R. (1965). *Transformations*. London: Karnac.

Bion, W.R. (1970). *Attention and Interpretation*. London: Tavistock (reprinted London: Karnac, 1984).

Bion, W.R. (1976). *Clinical Seminars and Other Works* (pp. 241–292). Abingdon: Fleetwood (reprinted London: Karnac, 1994].

Bion, W.R. (1980). *Bion in New York and Sao Paolo*. London: Karnac.

Bion, W.R. (1990). *Brazilian Lectures*. London: Karnac.

Chuster, A. (2014). *The Road not Taken*. Brazil: Trio Studio Bureau.

Chuster, A. (2018). Personal communication.

Chuster, A. (2019). Personal communication.

Grotstein, J. (2006). Personal communication.

Grotstein, J. S. (2007). *A Beam of Intense Darkness. Wilfred Bion's Legacy to Psychoanalysis.* London: Karnac.

Keats, John (1958). *Selected Letters of John Keats*, edited by G.F. Scott. Cambridge: Harvard University Press.

Meltzer, D., & Harris Williams, M. (1988). *The Apprehension of Beauty: The Role of Aesthetic Conflict in Development, Violence and Art.* Strath Tay: Clunie Press.

Sandler, P.C. (2005). *The Language of Bion: A Dictionary of Concepts.* London: Karnac.

Index

Abel-Hirsch, Nicola 8
achievement, language of 11–12, 114, **143**, 154–155, 158
action 56–57, 61, 93; language as 98; and negative capability 154–155, 158
adolescence, theory of 15
aesthetic dimension 63–64, 108–109, 117, 164
Aisenstein, M. 101n10
Alisobhani, Afsaneh Kiany 5, 11–12, 47
All My Sins Remembered: Another Part of a Life (Bion) 2–3, 19
alpha dreamwork 109, 111–112, 118
alpha elements 98–99, 107, 109, 111
alpha function 6, 17, 32, 46, 49, 98; and reverie of analyst 107, 110, 115; somato-psychic 110–111
Amiens, battle of (August 8, 1918) 1
analyst: anxiety of contact with patient 112–113; arrogance of 3–4; and beta screen 99–100; conundrum of 31–32, 35–36; curiosity of 3–4, 31, 36; free-floating attention required of 103–105, 109, 117; frustration in 83–86, 87, 89; knowingness (K and O) 39, 68; memory and desire, avoidance of 105–106, 112–115; mental state of during session 103; O as mental discipline for 9–10; as "obstructive object" 4, 32, 33–34, 38–39, 49, 76; O of 12, 74–75; as own psychic object 110; as poet 154; psychotic part within 63–64, 65–66; pursuit of knowledge and truth at all costs 3, 31; receptivity and metabolizing function 32; and reverie 107–110; understanding, letting go of 113

analytic session: delusion created by 124–125; free-floating attention in 103–105, 109, 117; here and now of 10, 36, 105, 115–116, 130–131; and reverie 107–110; transformation of the analytic experience 137. *See also* analyst; language; patient (analysand)
annihilation anxiety 93
anticipatory thinking 62, 66–67
a priori 47, 57
A-Santamaría Psychoanalysis Mexico A.C. 1
"attacks on linking" 43, 52, 59, 62, 80, 87, 125
attention: and consciousness 92; "free-floating" 103–105, 109, 117; and memory 92–93
Attention and Interpretation (Bion) 6, 7, 9, 11, 36, 91–102, 113, 153
autobiography 16–17; parallel autobiographical process 26–27; psychoanalytic 17; survivor subgenre 16–17
autopoiesis 66

Bacon, Francis 121
"bad object" 45–46, 94
being and being-there 11
Bergstein, Avner 10, 98
beta elements 6, 95, 98–99, 107; "idées mères" 111
beta screen 99–100
binocular vision 6, 109, 124, 154–155
Bion, Wilfred: authorial performativity 18; autobiographical narratives 2–3, 16–17; at boarding school 15–27; childhood and adolescence 15–16; developments in technique 115–117;